How Will They Know If I'm

Dead?

Transcending Disability and Terminal Illness

How Will They Know If I'm

Dead?

Transcending Disability
and Terminal Illness

Robert C. Horn, III

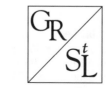

GR/St. Lucie Press
Delray Beach, Florida

Back cover photograph by Ricardo De Aratanha, *Los Angeles Times*.

Direct all inquires to: GR Press/St. Lucie Press, Inc., 100 E. Linton Blvd., Suite 403B, Delray Beach, Florida 33483. Phone: (561) 274-9906 or Fax (561) 274-9927.

Published by
GR Press/St. Lucie Press
100 E. Linton Blvd., Suite 403B
Delray Beach, FL 33483

Especially to Judy

Contents

About the Author ix

Foreword by C. Everett Koop, M.D., Sc.D. xi

Preface by David Richardson xiii

Acknowledgments xv

Introduction xvii

Part One: Living Life 1

    Chapter 1   Prelude to a Decision 3

    Chapter 2   Attitude Adjustment 13

Part Two: Choosing Life 17

    Chapter 3   Dealing with the Downhill 19

    Chapter 4   This is the Good News? 33

    Chapter 5   Coping I: Amazing Technology 37

    Chapter 6   Coping II: Wondrous People 51

Part Three: Affirming Life 61

    Chapter 7   Shift Change! 63

    Chapter 8   Reaching without Arms 77

In Place of a Conclusion 95

    Getting On with the Business of Living 97

Appendix 103

Selected, Annotated Bibliography 141

About the Author

Robert C. Horn, III is Professor Emeritus of Political Science at California State University, Northridge. His areas of specialization are the Soviet Union/Russia and international conflict resolution. He and his wife, Judy, a pre-school director, live in Los Angeles. They have three grown children, two of whom are currently living in Japan and one in Colorado. The entire family was active over the years in soccer, and Bob was instrumental in bringing girls soccer to the Los Angeles school system. Among Bob's favorite activities are reading, writing a monthly column for his church newsletter, and managing *Da Slugs*, his fantasy baseball team.

Foreword

I've known Robert Horn all his life, and I've learned a lot from him. From the time he was born, just about the time when my first son was born, I knew him as Robbie. My son and Robbie played together as toddlers, and then followed similar paths to academic careers, active sports, and family life. But then, with alarming suddenness, Robert's path through life took a startling change. In 1988, he, like many others in many other circumstances, was forced to hear the chilling words of a grim diagnosis. A series of bothersome but apparently innocuous symptoms turned out to be ALS — amyotrophic lateral sclerosis, more commonly known as Lou Gerhig's disease. ALS is a degenerative neuromuscular disease that quickly denies its victims voluntary muscle control, including the muscles needed to breathe. ALS is a terrible disease, and while it exacts its deadly toll from the body, it does not affect the mind. Its victims are completely aware of their continued and relentless physical degeneration. All too soon, ALS victims become unable to move, unable to speak above a strained whisper, unable to eat without choking, and barely able to breathe. ALS is a terminal disease, progressive and merciless. People with ALS don't usually live very long, the average life expectancy after diagnosis is two to four years.

But Robert Horn has lived longer than that already. And Robert Horn has truly LIVED. Even while afflicted with this deadly crippling disease, Robert has done more real living than most of us ever do. Many in his condition would find it difficult to face life. Most people find it difficult to face death. Every day, Robert Horn faces life and death at the same time; he faces life and death with joy, grace, and triumph.

I've had my share of experiences with life and death issues throughout a medical career that has spanned over half a century. At about the time when I first met the newborn Robbie Horn, I and a few others were pioneers in the new field of pediatric surgery, attempting to give years of life to those newborns whose serious congenital defects then had a mortality rate of 90%. By the time I left my surgical career nearly 40 years later, we had converted that 90% mortality rate into a 90% survival rate. Modern medicine can do great things, but modern medicine cannot do everything, as the grim course of ALS reminds us. But all those tiny lives we saved as surgeons — as important as each one was — were fewer in number than the many lives I saw changed when I served as United States Surgeon General, lives saved, not by medical miracles, but by individual choices: choices not to smoke, choices to quit smoking, choices to practice healthful living.

Robert Horn as chosen life — faced with the choice between death and a life all too many would say was not worth living. Robert chose life, and in doing so he has made so many of us realize anew how much life is worth living. He could easily have chosen another way; he was offered the option of ending his life painlessly and quickly. Instead he chose life, even life on a ventilator, "eating" through a tube inserted in his stomach, "talking" with his eyebrows, writing on a computer with his foot. Did he make the right choice? Robert's words bear repeating: "You bet! I am convinced that what I have left is more valuable than what I have lost. I believe that the things I can do are more important than those I can't. There is much more to life than physical ability. I am still a vibrant, healthy, and independent person mentally, emotionally, and spiritually. I can think, reason, and analyze, remember, read, write, learn and communicate. I can love, feel happiness and sadness, be enthusiastic, get angry, have highs and lows, feel joy. I can believe, hope, and have faith."

By God's grace, Robert lives a life of faith, hope, and love. And because he faces life and death with joy, grace, and triumph, I think you will, too, as you read his book.

by C. Everett Koop, M.D., Sc.D.

Preface

"The Courage to Be"

Years ago, I read Paul Tillich's book, *The Courage to Be.* It was one of the formative books of my life, certainly my intellectual life. Tillich's analysis of anxiety and faith is brilliant. His recollection of Kierkegaard and the existentialist's understanding of the way death impacts the psyche has fully informed my work as a pastor and my own inner struggles with life. What I have learned from books, however, has come nowhere close to what I have learned from Bob Horn, who has had to live out the crises that the philosophers and psychologists write about. In living with ALS, Bob has illustrated to everyone who knows him the power of faith and the meaning of courage. He does this simply and without much philosophizing or deep inner revelations. Perhaps this is what is so remarkable about this book. It is so straightforward, so natural, and so very much Bob Horn. Few people understand how he can endure so much. The heart of his power is an amazing gift of acceptance and recognition of destiny rather than resignation to fate.

In his journal, Kierkegaard wrote, "There is a world of difference between the proud courage which dares to fear the worst and the humble courage which dares to hope for the best." From the moment that Bob heard that terrible word "ALS" (Lou Gehrig's disease), he had no choice but to fear the worst, yet in his humble way he always hoped for the best. Torn between these two emotions, fear and hope, Bob endured the many months of testing and mixed diagnoses. He chose intentionally not to know more than he needed to about fearful things. This was not denial but a deliberate attempt to avoid the lure of succumbing to predictions. As a social scientist Bob knew the power of self-fulfilling prophecy. By choosing what he could handle, Bob managed to carry this awful burden a little load at a time, thus leaving energy to keep on with his teaching, his coaching, his friendships, and his joy. To outsiders it seemed almost too easy. How can he do it? Only Bob and those closest him know that it was not easy, but even they wonder how he did it. He has managed to squeeze out of life the maximum of joy, accomplishment, and happiness in spite of the most limiting circumstances. He has indeed had the courage to *be* despite the threat of non-being. This book is his story told in his own way about the inimical circumstances that life presented him these past years. Bob, however, has made peace even with this. He has made a friend of his adversary. As Hemingway put it, "Courage is grace under pressure." In Bob Horn, all of us who know him, have experienced grace in a new way.

David Richardson
Pastor, Northridge United Methodist Church
June 1995

ACKNOWLEDGEMENTS

"You should write a book."

If I had a penny for every time someone has said that to me over the past few years, I bet I'd have at least a dollar! Maybe even a buck-fifty!

Such suggestions, however, are no justification for actually sitting down at the word processor and pounding, or kicking in my case (on that, more later), one out. Besides, I had already written a book — albeit a very different kind, an academic study of relations between the Soviet Union and India — and knew the enormous amount of work involved. Writing is not sitting at the typewriter on the balcony of a cabin in the mountains with a glass of scotch in hand. (Some of you may remember that idyllic scene in ads for a particular brand of scotch.) At least, it wasn't that way for me earlier and it certainly isn't that way now. For me, writing is extremely rewarding work, but it is still work.

The bottom line is that you better have something of interest and/or importance to say. If you don't, it is not worth writing; if it is written, it is not worth publishing; and, if it happens to be published, it won't be worth reading.

I believe I have something to say. Almost as important, people who know me and have read the articles about my situation and outlook think so, too. It is those folks to whom I owe heartfelt gratitude for encouraging me to collect my thoughts and organize them in written form. Many of them have also provided invaluable assistance to this project. Even so, they all refuse to assume any of the responsibility for shortcomings or errors, insisting that I shoulder that alone. Imagine that?! Unable to spread the blame, I am forced to acquiesce.

The shortlist of people who have been major sources of encouragement and assistance begins with my family, wife Judy, sons Jeff and Chris, and daughter Laura. The list also includes my close friend David Stowe; my brother Dr. Thomas Horn, a psychiatrist and Associate Chief of Clinical Services at the Western Psychiatric Institute and Clinic, University of Pittsburgh Medical Center; my good friend and pastor Dr. David Richardson, Senior Minister of Northridge United Methodist Church; my mother, Dorothy Horn; my late aunt, Eleanor Horn; my physician Dr. Gordon Dowds; and Gretchen Keeler, who has been my Administrative Assistant since 1989.

The crucial factors in my ability to deal with my disability and disease have been the love, support, and generosity of family and friends. This is a very long list. I can't possibly thank all of them by name. Inasmuch as they are also the ones who are really responsible for this book, it is dedicated to them and to the countless people who are fighting their own battles against a debilitating, life-threatening, or terminal illness.

INTRODUCTION

I coached youth soccer for 15 years and I absolutely loved it. Eleven of those years I coached my daughter and the girls, from five- and six-year-old kids who were just beginning the sport all the way through city champion high schoolers and exceptionally talented under-16 and under-19 club teams. I love the game — the exercise, fun and, especially, the necessity of teamwork. Most of all, I loved the kids. I coached a lot of the girls for many years and got to know them and their families very well. They became almost daughters to me. "My girls" I proudly called them and they were and still are special young ladies.

I approached coaching as another form of teaching. Just as I was a professor in the classroom, I was a teacher on the soccer field. Further, I also was convinced that a person who takes on the responsibility of coaching young people has an obligation to try to teach them more than the mechanics of that particular sport. Being entrusted with these youth for even a few hours each week is a great privilege and the opportunity to pass along some "life lessons" should not be missed. Like it or not, for better or worse, a coach is a role model and his/her attitude toward the game and toward life can have a significant impact on a youngster's outlook. So, one's influence had better be a positive one.

With all of these considerations in mind, and being careful not to intrude into the realm of parental authority, the coaches I worked with and I emphasized a few basic principles that apply not only to soccer but also to the broader concerns of life. For instance, we stressed sportsmanship, fair play, hard work, self-confidence, and respect for teammates and opponents. Simple precepts but fundamental, I think, to any endeavor and to that old-fashioned idea of "character."

As the girls grew older, I became a bit more philosophical. Impressed with the concept of the game of soccer as a metaphor for life, I developed a little homily that became an integral part of my pre-game oratory. In its full version, it went something like this: "Soccer is like life. It doesn't matter how often you get knocked down or if you lose the ball or make a mistake. Those things happen to each of us. What does matter is whether and how quickly you recover, learn from the experience, and get back in the game. That's the test of character."

Somehow, when you are delivering such inspirational pronouncements, you are not thinking of yourself but, rather, in terms of your audience. At least, that was true in my case. In my life, after all, I had had to overcome setbacks, disappointments, and my own mistakes but, thankfully, none of them had been major or life-threatening. So it was that I was unprepared to apply my little bit of homespun philosophy to my own life in a big-time way.

All that changed on one sunny Friday afternoon in June 1988: I was given a death sentence.

On that horrific day, I was told that I had Lou Gehrig's disease, known medically as Amyotrophic Lateral Sclerosis or ALS. The diagnosis came out of the blue. I went into the neurologist's office with a minor twitch in my left arm and came out with a fatal motor neuron disease. My world was suddenly turned upside-down. ALS is a particularly nasty disease that kills you gradually, progressively, by blocking the messages from the brain to the muscles. Within just a few years, often less than two, the muscles atrophy to the point of total paralysis. This paralysis includes the muscles that control swallowing and, most essential to life, breathing. Basically, death is by suffocation. ALS leaves the mind intact so it can observe this steady physical deterioration.

The statistics regarding ALS are as grisly and despair-inducing as the disease itself. No one survives it. It is terminal in all cases. A small percentage of its victims live for 10 years and an even smaller number live for 20 years (British scientist Stephen Hawking is probably the best-known example) but ALS always wins. The overriding, and overwhelming, statistic is that the average life expectancy for an ALS victim is only three to five years from the time of the diagnosis. Some sources put it at two to four years.

I was not a quantitative political scientist when I was teaching at the university and I am no whiz at statistics, but it seems to me that, judging from the above numbers, I should be dead. In fact, by the "law" of statistical probability, I should have died several years ago!

Perhaps that's why I distrust statistics. Except in sports, especially baseball. In baseball, statistics tell all — actually, they don't in "real" baseball but they do in "fantasy" baseball. I have had a team in a fantasy league for as long as I have had ALS and every morning for the last seven seasons I have poured over box scores to see how various members of my team — Da Slugs — performed in five batting and five pitching categories. Their aggregate statistics determine everything.

In sum, from my perspective, baseball statistics are almost sacred, fit to be carved in stone. Statistics about ALS, on the other hand, are best ignored. To the extent that such negative statistics can become self-fulfilling prophecies, they are to be doubly ignored.

Moreover, the fact of the matter is that I am just too busy living to pay much attention to ALS mortality statistics.

Most of the books I have read about ALS and other terminal illnesses are understandably focused mostly on dying and death. This book is not mainly about either. Nor, as you might guess, does it deal with statistics. There are hardly any numbers in it at all. It is not about the medical aspects of ALS or other crippling and terminal diseases. Nor is it a compilation of the experiences of various people dealing with ALS or anything else. Finally, it is not by a celebrity author about his recent illness and recovery.

What this book is about, then, is living. It is about life. First and foremost, it is about the value and rewards of living life to the fullest extent possible in spite of being under the shadow of a terminal disease and having severe disabilities. It is about coping, about perseverance and determination, and, ultimately, about hope. It is a story of one person's struggle. It is a personal celebration of the triumph of life over disease and death.

The book, like Caesar's Gaul, is divided into three parts. Part One, "Living Life," sets the stage for my confrontation with ALS. First, it presents some personal background which is intended to give the reader an idea of how much I enjoyed my "previous life" and where, literally, I am coming from. Second, it discusses my attitude toward, well...attitude. "Choosing Life," Part Two, focuses on my struggle with the disease, the extraordinary support I received in those difficult times, my decision in favor of life and the means of coping with my new situation. Part Three, "Affirming Life," discusses the fragility of life when you are dependent on others for survival and also reflects on what I gratefully consider to be my new lease on life. The "nonconclusion" attempts to tie the remaining loose ends together.

I have been coping, battling if you prefer, with ALS for just over seven years now. I have had virtually no functioning muscles for five years. I can't eat, speak, or move. And I have been hooked to a ventilator for the past four-and-a-half years. That machine breathes for me. Everything I do takes a great deal of time. Communicating is especially slow. I "speak" with my eyebrows and spelling out every word letter by letter is a tedious and lengthy process. About five hours of each of my days are consumed by necessary medical attention, getting bathed and dressed, taking a nap and, finally, being transported out to the living room where my computer waits with considerably more patience than its eager user. On my good days, I am usually able to work for five to six hours before I get too tired. I type with the only part of my body that I can move, my right foot, and this is another slow process. It takes me, on average, almost two days to type a page. Everything is a project.

What, then, is my message? It is simply this: I have found, along with many others, that despite the difficult conditions of disability and terminal illness, life can be meaningful, productive, fulfilling, rewarding, and valuable.

PART ONE

LIVING LIFE

1

PRELUDE TO A DECISION

I have no complaints about my life. I have, luckily, only a few regrets and none of them is of cosmic significance. In fact, prior to ALS, I loved my life!

I grew up into my mid-forties a very normal person and yet, at the same time, a somewhat abnormal one. I was normal in the sense that there was nothing particularly unusual about me, no involvement in anything, positive or negative, unique or spectacular. I was, I think, abnormal in the abundance of blessings and joys I have received. I thoroughly enjoyed, and appreciated, my family, my job, my other activities, and my friends. I have lived a wonderful life and consider myself an extremely fortunate man.

Growing Up Normal

I am tempted to say that "I grew up a poor, black child" but that was Steve Martin's line in his (classically bad?) movie *The Jerk*. It wouldn't be true, in any case. Actually, I grew up a WASP — white, Anglo-Saxon, Protestant — and middle-class. I wasn't even a latchkey kid. My mother was a housewife who did a lot of volunteer work but always made sure she was there when I got home from school. My father was a physician, a professor of pathology at the medical school of the University of Pennsylvania. I had a very happy and secure childhood, marred only by chronic, periodically acute, asthma. My brother Tom and sister Ethel, both younger, and I were neither indulged nor deprived.

Evidently, I was not always as pleasant and charming as I would like to think of myself now. For instance, I can't imagine it but my family contends that I, unjustly I am sure, spent the most time in the infamous and dreaded "Big Puss Chair." That chair was the place of banishment for anyone of, so to say, "displeasing disposition." Talking back and being generally obnoxious periodically seem to have been my preferred means of "getting the Chair." Fortunately, this seat of discipline was located not in Philadelphia but in Maine — on a beautiful mountain-surrounded lake where Tom, Ethel, and I would spend a glorious month swimming, fishing, boating, playing in the woods, and trying, unsuccessfully almost every time, to make popcorn by shaking a long-handled basket over the fire — so it was not a permanent threat.

(To remind me of this lesson in humility, my sister and her husband, Kim, had a large charcoal drawing made from an old photograph showing me slumped, with the appropriate sour countenance, in the chair. The drawing is very well done and hangs in our family room.)

There were several benchmark events or turning points in my early life. One of them was our move to Detroit in 1955. Grosse Pointe Park, where we lived, had a superb school system. I prospered academically all the way through high school. I not only learned how to learn but I also developed a genuine love for and joy in, as well as a sense of satisfaction from, learning. Two sports were my favorite recreational activities. A group of us played backyard basketball almost daily — usually at my house because, with the help of brickwork between the garage doors, we could dunk. And, after taking lessons, I spent whole days playing tennis. In addition to learning, both became lifelong passions and pleasures.

Baseball became another such passion. This was not so much to play, although I ended up playing a good deal of softball, as to watch and appreciate. In short, I became a fan. I have my Dad to thank for this. He took me to my first Phillies games when I was young and his love for the "national pastime" was contagious. In my high school years and thereafter I spent countless happy hours in the bleachers at Tiger Stadium and Boston's Fenway Park, and even Yankee and Shea Stadiums when I was in New York. Once my own children were old enough, I began to take them to Dodger Stadium partly because I loved it and partly because I wanted them to love it, too. They do.

Choosing Wittenberg University in Ohio for college proved to be another benchmark event. Wittenberg is a small, liberal arts, Lutheran church-related school with an excellent undergraduate program. My four years there were full of tremendous personal growth — intellectual, emotional, and social (which is just what the college experience is supposed to be). I was exposed to several gifted teachers, particularly in political science and American history. They were responsible for triggering my interest in teaching as a career. I joined a good fraternity and was active in student government, learning some invaluable leadership skills and certain equally valuable truths about politics.

Among all the contributions Wittenberg made to my life, the most significant was Judy Eppers, my future wife. We started dating in our senior year and pretty soon fell in love with each other. By graduation, in June of 1964, we both knew it was for real and we planned the next year accordingly. Since I had a choice of graduate schools of international relations and Judy was going to be in New York City, I was able to opt for my first preference, The Fletcher School of Law and Diplomacy just outside Boston. The vast majority of weekends found one of us aboard a Greyhound bus headed either to New York or Boston. It was a good year, full of sightseeing and Broadway shows (including Barbra Streisand in *Funny Girl* and Zero Mostel in *Fiddler on the Roof*). Oh yes, I also did find some time to read and study.

However, we rapidly grew tired of long-distance romance (besides, Greyhound didn't have a Frequent Rider program) and we decided to get married sooner rather than later. We had a beautiful ceremony that August in Buffalo, Judy's hometown.

Judy worked as a secretary for the next two years to support us while I completed my coursework and began research for my Ph.D. dissertation on Soviet foreign policy toward Indonesia. I chose that topic because two professors, one a specialist on the Soviet Union and the other on Asia, through their knowledge and teaching skill opened up these fascinating worlds to me. Both continue to excite my interest.

Parochial to Global (Around the World in 365 Days)

Now for some distinct abnormality. Or just plain good fortune. This choice of a thesis topic had a serendipitous effect as well. It seems that a donor of fellowships for dissertation research in Third World countries was deluged with applications for Africa and Latin America but was looking for worthwhile Asian ones. I had the right topic at the right time! I was granted a fellowship to conduct research in Indonesia!

The grant included a $4,000 stipend and round-trip airfare for me. Since Detroit, our point of departure, was on the opposite side of the world from Jakarta, Indonesia's capital, a round-the-world ticket, valid for a year, was the same price as a round-trip one (about $1,200). Guess which we chose? After we paid for Judy's ticket out of our so-called savings, we were faced with the reality of having to live on my stipend for the year. In 1967-68, however, that was possible, provided you weren't too choosy about where you stayed or what you ate. Especially where you stayed. We weren't and we made it through the year with a few dozen dollars to spare.

And what a fantastic year it was! We traveled through East Asia for a month on our way to Indonesia, lived there for seven months, and then took four months getting home via more of Asia, the Middle East, and Eastern and Western Europe. The highlights are too numerous to mention. For someone whose previous international travel consisted of Canada (Judy had been to Europe) and who wanted to teach about international relations, it was an extraordinary education.

Living in Indonesia, in particular, was invaluable for both of us in many ways. Unfortunately, gathering concrete data for my dissertation was not one of them. We were there just two years after the crushing of a Communist-backed coup attempt and absolutely no one wanted to talk about any sort of Communist, whether they be local or Chinese or Soviet. Nor did organized archives exist. I did talk with and get to know many Russians, interviewed some relevant people, and gathered a small handful of useful documentary material. The overriding value of my time in Indonesia was the "feel" I got for the country and its diverse peoples, its many cultures, and its foreign policy perspectives. This made me a better teacher and better scholar.

An unexpected benefit of the lack of data was that it freed us to get out into the country beyond the capital city and its immediate environs; we spent nearly three months traveling through the cultural centers and rural areas of the main island of Java, Bali, and Sumatra. Indonesia's myriad differences from what we were used to were exceedingly fascinating and instructive.

The year was, in sum, an education.

My Professional Niche

As you might expect, we came home from our year two very changed people, our perspectives broadened and our sensitivities sharpened. The return to Fletcher would have been completely anticlimactic had it not been for three goals we had firmly in mind: for me to finish my dissertation, for me to get a teaching job, and for us to start a family.

Cutting to the chase, in September 1969 we found ourselves in a new city, a new state, with two new jobs, and with a new baby. I had finished my dissertation and successfully defended it and managed to obtain one of the increasingly scarce college teaching positions. As an Assistant Professor of Political Science at San Fernando Valley State College — soon renamed California State University, Northridge — just "over the hill" from Los Angeles, I was teaching my specialty, Soviet foreign policy, and earning what seemed to us to be a princely sum of almost $11,000(!).

I quickly realized that teaching was where I belonged, my niche. It played to my aptitudes and strengths as well as the opportunity for growth, both in skills in the classroom and professionally as a scholar. I loved everything, except grading, about my job, especially the constant intellectual stimulation I got from colleagues and students. Every day was different, with new challenges, opportunities and, usually, rewards. I enjoyed my students and cared about the ones I was able to get to know. Moreover, I also thought I was doing in an important way — contributing to the future.

My most enjoyable teaching experiences were with the simulations, or role-playing exercises, I developed as a learning tool in most of my classes. These usually worked well in engaging students, getting them to be active participants in the learning process, which was my primary objective. They taught them, in a very personal way, about perception and perspective which are central to the understanding of politics on any level.   Some of the simulations were rather ambitious, like the one I did with another professor on Soviet and American crisis decisionmaking. But the most ambitious, and arguably the most successful, was the Model United Nations program. It was a year-long course that "trained" — on the country, the issues involved, and diplomatic strategies and skills — the students to represent an assigned country at an annual conference of scores of universities and colleges. It was an amazing learning experience. It also had an additional benefit: it brought a group of students together in a way unusual for a large and partly commuter school like Northridge.

I became convinced early on that research, whether for presentation to professional meetings, publication, or personal use, is an integral part of teaching at the college level. At least, I know it is for me. I began to write papers for regional Slavic, Asian, and international studies organizations. Almost all of them were published in various professional journals. This was the beginning of a nearly 20-year "career" of activity in the profession, participating in regional, national, and international conferences and publishing more than two dozen articles, numerous book reviews, several chapters in edited books, a couple of monographs, and one book. Judy and I finally got abroad again in 1979 as a result of one of those international meetings. We spent three weeks in the Soviet Union, mainly in Central Asia, before I attended the International Political Science Association conference in Moscow. Over the next few years I had meetings in West Germany, Japan, Taiwan, and France.

Just For Kicks

In 1977, I discovered an avocation — coaching youth soccer. Although I became involved quite by accident, I quickly came to love it and coached for the next 15 years. Jeff, who was very athletic, started when he was six at a park just down the street. He loved it from the first kick. The experience for equally athletic Chris, however, was not so positive. In fact, he didn't want to play again after his first year; he simply hadn't enjoyed it, mainly because of a less than competent coach whose entire philosophy of coaching seemed to consist of screeching "Pass it to Jason" (her son). Chris and I agreed that soccer should be fun. I was convinced that, under the right circumstances, he would love the sport as his brother did so I offered to coach his team the following year, try to make it fun, and if he still didn't enjoy it, we would both retire. Chris accepted, I spent most of my summer reading soccer books and, as the cliché goes, the rest is history. He and I loved it!

SALLY FORTH By Greg Howard and Craig MacIntosh

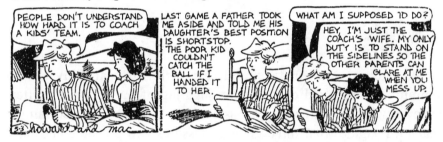

Reprinted with special permission of King Features Syndicate.

I coached Chris for three years before deciding it was time for him to experience other, more knowledgeable coaches. By then, however, I was hooked so I started coaching Laura, then age six, and the girls. (Since she was our youngest, she got stuck with me for a long time.) We thoroughly enjoyed each year and did very well. My friend Bill Daws and I took teams to all-star and other tournaments all over Southern California, to Tucson, and to Hawaii all under the auspices of the American Youth Soccer Organization. Then we formed a club team and continued to play in leagues and travel to tournaments (including a big national one, which we won, in Colorado Springs). We were an excellent team and, just as importantly, we all had a terrific time, the girls, the coaches, and the parents.

I am very proud of the role I played, along with many others, in finally persuading officials of the Los Angeles Unified School District to make girls soccer an interscholastic sport in the fall of 1988. In the spring of the following year, I was honored to be asked to coach the girls team at Chatsworth High School where our boys had gone and Laura was to be a sophomore; it seems that the first-year coach didn't work out, despite the fact that the girls won the first of five consecutive city championships for the school. With the crucial assistance of my long-time friend Jack Sidwell, now the head coach, and Steve Berk, a friend and a PE teacher at the school, I was able to coach the team for two years before ALS, which had slowed me, then finally stopped me altogether. I loved those two years!

Family Matters

My teaching and professional responsibilities and my soccer commitments required considerable juggling of my schedule. Often, however, what took precedence was neither of these but, rather, family. I cannot imagine what three greater blessings two people could have than three healthy, happy children. I knew how fortunate I was and I was determined to miss as little as possible of their growing up.

Our family definitely had top priority every summer. Judy and I wanted our children to know their grandparents, aunts, uncles, and cousins. We thought — and are convinced now — that they would greatly benefit from a strong sense of family just as we had. My schedule allowed us to have extended visits with both of our families every summer. Even after I taught a course or two in summer school, we would still have six or seven weeks for our trip "back East." We drove (except when the first of two engine fires in our otherwise beloved VW camper encouraged us, temporarily, to enjoy the comforts of Amtrak), usually camped, often visited friends and historical sites, and always stopped in Denver to see Judy's sister, Marcia, and her brother, Jim, and their families. Our stay with my parents invariably included a Tigers game and a wonderful two or three days fishing at a beautiful and tranquil trout club in northern Ohio. Judy's parents had a cottage on a lovely bay of Lake Erie, just south of Buffalo, where Judy (and her mother) spent all of her summers. There we would swim, boat, fish, play tennis, golf, and bridge, among other activities. We also saw Judy's brother, Don, who lived in Buffalo and my brother, Tom, in Pittsburgh and both of their families. That meant our children saw all of their immediate relatives on a regular basis, with the exception of my sister and her family; Ethel lived "off" any of our routes East or West but we did make it up to her home in Juneau, Alaska, one summer. We all loved our summer vacations of traveling, playing and enjoying family. It was for us, as in Fiddler on the Roof, a very important tradition.

One international experience the entire family participated in was a year in the Southeast Asian country of Malaysia in 1983-84. I was awarded a Fulbright Visiting Professorship at two universities on the outskirts of Kuala Lumpur, Malaysia's capital city, the University of Malaya and The National University (UKM). We lived in a nice house in a lovely faculty housing area adjacent to the University of Malaya campus. The kids, now in ninth, seventh, and fourth grades, all went to the International School of Kuala Lumpur. ISKL was a wonderful school, not only because of the high quality of its teaching but also because children from almost 50 countries attended it. Talk about a multicultural experience! Moreover, Malaysia has a great deal of its own to offer. It is a fascinating mosaic of ethnic and cultural diversity. We got to know many interesting and gracious people and were able to witness, and often share in, various Malay, Chinese and Indian festivals and celebrations. We also took advantage of Malaysia's many holidays and traveled all over the country. When we weren't traveling, I divided my time between teaching, research, and coaching assorted sports teams at the kids' school. Judy helped at the school, ran the Girl Scouts and, among other activities, had a cooking group with three friends, Malaysian, Japanese, and Australian. All in all, it was an incredible year — including the trip home via Singapore, Indonesia, Hong Kong, and Japan — a real eye-opener for our kids and a great education for each of us.

I hope it is now clear why I said at the beginning of this chapter that my life has been one rich in blessings. And, as you know, the joy is in the myriad details of life which I could only hint at in this sketch. Some may call it being lucky or fortunate but I prefer to call it being blessed. I am thankful, too, that I realized much of it at the time. I thanked God often for His abundant gifts.

In spite of difficulties, the blessings continued. They continue to this day.

2

ATTITUDE ADJUSTMENT

In our contemporary society, how many of us feel in control of our lives? I would venture to say that most of us feel that our lives, totally or in part, are beyond our control. Life happens TO us. Most of the time we are forced to react rather than act. Things happen too fast, the pace of life is too hectic, technology too complex, finances confusing, and on and on. Despite all our scrambling to keep up, many, if not most, of us seem to be falling further behind.

Multiply this feeling of loss of control by a factor of, say, 100 and you can approach an understanding of the perspective of people with disabilities or life-threatening illnesses. This is especially true in the initial period as the person gropes to make sense of what has happened and to comprehend what it means for the future. This helpless feeling of having no control over what happens to you is a constant companion of the disabled and particularly those with life-threatening or terminal illnesses.

To quote the founder of the late and unlamented Soviet Union, Vladimir Lenin, "What is to be done?" Clearly, the loss of control must be struggled against. The afflicted person must try to regain some measure of control over his or her life. But that is far easier said than done. Is there anything at all a person, afflicted or not, can control? As a matter of fact, there is — our mental outlook, our attitude.

I receive a variety of publications, including reports, newsletters, research updates, articles, etc., from various branches of the ALS and Muscular Dystrophy Associations. Usually, the most thought-provoking to me are the personal perspectives by people with one of the diseases. In a recent packet from the Michigan ALS chapter I found a brief article by a Charles Swindoll which was excerpted from another ALS chapter's publication. It is entitled "Attitude" and it struck a responsive chord in me. I think it also is applicable to anyone, handicapped or not. (This was confirmed by the enthusiastic reception of dozens of people when I included it in an article I wrote for our church newsletter.)

Mr. Swindoll writes:

> "The longer I live, the more I realize the impact of attitude on life. To me, attitude is more important than facts. It is more important than the past, than education, than money, than circumstances, than failures, than successes, than what other people think or say or do. It is more important than appearance, giftedness or skill. It will make or break a company, a church, a home.
>
> "The remarkable thing is we have a choice every day, regarding the attitude we will embrace for that day. We cannot change our past. We cannot change the fact that people will act in a certain way. We cannot change the inevitable. The only thing we can do is play on the one string we have, and that is our attitude. . . . I am convinced that life is 10% what happens to me and 90% how I react to it."

I think he hit the nail squarely on the head. The simple fact is that we cannot control external events or forces. That is the reality. But another part of that reality is that we do have control over how we react to what happens to us. Our attitude is of enormous significance and should not be underestimated.

This is not meant to imply that attitude can alter the nature and course of disease. Or can it? There is a heated debate about this in the scientific literature. There seems to be an emerging consensus that social support, as opposed to social isolation, positively correlates to longevity in terminally ill patients. Much less agreement exists about the role of other psychological variables. Disease cannot be simply wished away by a positive attitude, but numerous recent studies have demonstrated a link between attitude and survival rates. For instance, people who are defiant and "battle" their disease have been shown to live longer than those who just give up.

One very interesting study along these lines which examined ALS patients was recently completed. It monitored the survival status of 144 volunteers for three-and-a-half years. At the beginning, researchers tested their subjects on a range of psychological variables and then divided them into three groups based on such factors as depression, hopelessness, and perceived stress. The findings are instructive. Of the group with the highest degrees of these factors, the highest level of psychological distress, 82% died within the time span of the study. In the middle group, 65% died. In the group with the lowest level of distress, however, only 32% died!

(Another study that I found particularly intriguing suggested that just having "an attitude" is good for you. Researchers at the Johns Hopkins Medical School divided women with breast cancer into two groups based on length of survival. They discovered that the long survivors were considered less cooperative by the hospital staff. Right on!)

Even more important, I think, is the impact of attitude on the quality of life. That is really the point and, on this, there is no substantial argument. The mind and body are closely intertwined. This relationship and its effect on health and quality of life are persuasively presented by Dr. David Spiegel in his book *Living Beyond Limits*. His conclusion, like Mr. Swindoll's and mine, is that a positive attitude can greatly enhance the quality of one's life.

If nothing else, as a Hallmark greeting card sent me by my friend Rosalyn (the church secretary!) said, "A positive attitude may not solve all your problems but it will annoy enough people to make it worth the effort." That, alone, should count for something.

PART TWO

CHOOSING LIFE

3

DEALING WITH THE DOWNHILL

The 1987-88 academic year was a truly outstanding one for me. It began with the award of a sabbatical for the fall semester. I was doing research on Soviet-Vietnamese relations in the hopes of expanding a monograph I had written on the subject (during a recent fellowship at the RAND Corporation) into a book. Thanks to Asian colleagues I met at a series of seminars at the East-West Center at the University of Hawaii, I was invited to speak and conduct interviews in several Asian countries. So Judy, who was not about to miss out on an excursion to Asia, and I made our first trip to China as well as return visits to Thailand, Singapore, Indonesia and, nostalgically, Malaysia. We saw many old friends and colleagues, met several new ones and I gathered a substantial amount of information and insights for my project. It was wonderful to be back in Asia and it was a terrific trip!

More special things happened in the spring semester. For one, our Model UN program made its long-discussed venture from the Far West regional conference to the National Conference in New York. That conference and that city have a number of advantages, particularly the actual United Nations and each country's official mission to the world body. The experience was so successful that, despite the additional fund-raising required, our program has participated in "nationals" ever since. At about the same time, I was informed that I was to be one of that year's recipients of the Distinguished Professor Award. I felt, and still feel, very honored by that award because it particularly recognizes teaching skills and success in the classroom. Finally, I spent almost two weeks in

Moscow in mid-May at the invitation of the Institute of Far Eastern Studies of the USSR Academy of Sciences. I did a seminar at that institute and had discussions with numerous scholars there and from other institutes. This visit was invaluable in bringing me up-to-date on evolving Soviet policy perspectives and giving me a first hand look at the exciting and monumental, and controversial, changes taking place under Gorbachev.

In other words, in the spring of 1988 I felt on top of the world. My life couldn't have been much better. Granted, I was not wealthy financially or in material terms but I considered myself rich in areas of far greater importance: family, religion, and employment. Judy and I had a loving and fulfilling marriage and our children (now in junior high, high school, and college) were doing well in all respects and continued to be a source of joy to us. We were active members of a dynamic Methodist church that more than met our spiritual needs, deepened our faith, and was filled with wonderful people. Finally, we both had jobs we enjoyed, college teaching in my case and directing a pre-school in Judy's, and that we felt made a contribution to the community. Professionally, my research was going very well.

So what was next? Immediately, there was another trip to Asia. I had arranged with the United States Information Agency to embark on a three-week speaking tour in Asia that summer under their auspices. The trip would include Australia and New Zealand, where I had never been, as well as Japan and would give me the opportunity of seeing a great many friends, personal and professional. I was eagerly looking forward to it.

The "roll" I was on was about to come to a sudden and devastating halt. The ancient Greeks said that "pride goeth before the fall." I don't really think my pride caused it but I was about to learn about the fall in a far too personal, firsthand and major way.

The Crash

After returning from Moscow, I spent most of my time in my tiny room in the campus library preparing my talks for the Asia trip. One day, early on, I noticed a very slight twitching in a muscle in my left arm, up near the shoulder. It was a little annoying and I tried, literally, to shake it off. That didn't work but I still didn't think much about it. Shortly thereafter, my daughter pointed out a similar twitching in my right thigh just above my knee. That was cause enough to force me, reluctantly, to schedule an appointment with my internist. He seemed stumped and, after several tests and a follow-up visit revealed nothing beyond the obvious and continuing twitching, he referred me to a neurologist.

The visit to the neurologist is, unfortunately, etched indelibly on my mind. (The only thing I can't recall is the name of the doctor; I suppose I have repressed it.) After he examined me, particularly checking my muscles and reflexes, he asked me what I thought might be the problem. "I don't know," I replied, still clueless. "A pinched nerve?" Then he said, with considerably more medical accuracy than bedside manner, "Have you ever heard of Lou Gehrig's disease?"

Of course I had; Gehrig was one of my baseball heroes. Then I went numb. The blood drained from my head, I couldn't finish getting dressed, and I had to lie down. There is no good way to deliver such news but his abrupt and harsh pronouncement was awful. The only "consolation" he could offer was that he would have to do a number of tests before a diagnosis could be confirmed.

It is still amazing to me how rapidly one can plummet from the heights of the mountaintop to the depths of the valley. Or at least how fast I could. And did. It was virtually instantaneous. One moment life was glorious and the next it appeared to be over. I knew what Lou Gehrig's disease meant: progressive loss of muscle control leading to death within a few, short, agonizing years. I was never going to be normal again. And, very soon I was going to die.

Dr. Elisabeth Kubler-Ross discusses coping with the news and reality of terminal illness in her excellent book *On Death and Dying*. She describes the various stages most people go through — indeed, must work through to arrive at an acceptance of the situation and get on with life. Another way of looking at the necessity of working through the psychological problems is the analogy of a swimmer caught in a riptide, as related to me by my pastor. You need to go with the force of it, not wasting your energy in a futile fight against it, and just ride it out. Only when its force is spent can you safely swim, sideways, to shore.

I am not a great swimmer in any case but I think I rode out that riptide of emotions fairly well. In retrospect, I also went through most, if not all, of the stages Kubler-Ross describes. They were not always in neat sequence but were often jumbled together. They also existed for varying periods.

For most of the first month I was in a state of shock and despair. I was devastated and seemed to alternate between listlessness and fidgety nervousness. These dominant emotions of despair and anxiety coincided with a version of her first stage, that of denial. It wasn't the traditional kind of denial, I don't think — I didn't insist that it couldn't be true, for example, but one born out of nature of the disease. There is no positive test or procedure for diagnosing ALS; it is "discovered" negatively, by testing for and eliminating other maladies. This doubt leads to a sort of hopeful denial. I canceled my Asia trip, underwent what seemed like at least 1,000 tests, including an update of one straight out of the Middle Ages involving needles and electrodes, and obtained a second opinion at Detroit's Henry Ford Hospital in this necessary process of elimination. I hoped, in vain, that some test or other would reveal that I had a less serious disease than ALS.

Simultaneous with this stage and extending somewhat beyond it was the anger stage. I was mad not at anyone or anything in particular but rather at my condition. For a time I was angry that this had happened to me. Why me and not someone else? I didn't deserve this! Fortunately, I was able to emerge from this stage fairly quickly.

I spent even less time in Kubler-Ross's third stage, bargaining. In fact, I am not sure I passed through this stage at all. Trying to make deals with God struck me as just about as productive as asking "Why did God do this to me ?" On the other hand, I did — and still do — think about what I would do with my life if I were suddenly, or gradually, cured and practical expressions of thanks to God figured prominently in each of my scenarios.

I did wallow in the depression stage for a bit longer. Looking back, this was the most necessary and important stage for me. It was the preparatory kind of depression, where one confronts the impending loss of people, places, and things he loves. (Actually, I think my situation fit better the definition of grief than that of depression. My "down" periods were frequent but of short duration and not really that deep. See Edgar Jackson, *Understanding Grief*, listed in the bibliography.) This was a very difficult time.

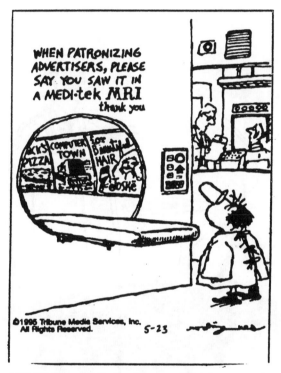

Have I now reached the fifth and final stage of acceptance? I think so, at least in most respects. I still have periods of being down in the dumps and occasionally being angry. These usually occur when I am particularly tired and, in any case, I suspect this is quite normal. Kubler-Ross defines the acceptance stage as being the absence of fear and despair. I am there.

Where I am confused, however, is with another part of her definition: she writes that acceptance also includes an acknowledgement that the struggle is over. Maybe I have misinterpreted her but my struggle is definitely not over. To paraphrase one of my favorite characters from, embarrassing though it may be to admit, one of my favorite movies, Bluto (played by the incomparable John Belushi) in *Animal House*, it ain't over until I say it's over. I refuse just to sit around waiting to die.

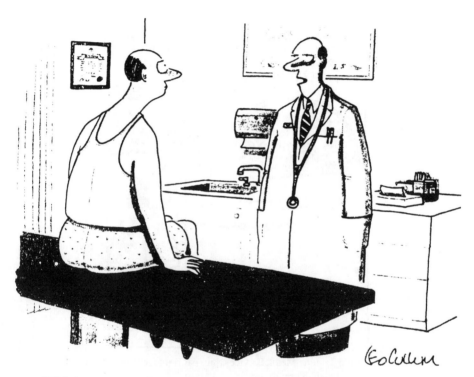

"This is a second opinion. At first, I thought you had something else."

Drawing by Cullum; ©1996 *The New Yorker Magazine*, Inc.

For me, every day is a struggle. I have always believed that being alive meant reaching, extending myself — not in a frantic manner but in a way that promotes continued growth, learning, expansion of my horizons, and the enrichment of my life and, I would be so presumptuous to hope, the lives of some others. This attitude is reinforced by the topic of Kubler-Ross's next chapter after the one on acceptance: hope. She doesn't list hope as a separate stage but an emotion accompanying all the stages. This is so important that it deserves a fuller treatment and I will return to it later.

In sum, I feel that I have achieved the stage of acceptance and the state of peace. But it is certainly not an acceptance or peace of resignation to my "fate." Rather, it is an acceptance and peace combined with a fighting spirit, a determination to make the most of what I have for as long as I have, and hope.

Searching

Not only did I run the gamut of emotions in the months following the diagnosis, I also went through my share of doctors, clinics, potential treatments, and experiments. With each, I unwisely got my hopes up. I was seen by neurologists and checked out in ALS clinics from Los Angeles to Detroit to Edmonton, Alberta, to San Diego. I participated in clinical trials and double-blind studies. Among other things, I injected myself with large doses of vitamin B, took increased quantities of other vitamins orally, and tried amino acids for quite a while (which also necessitated a substantial change in my diet).

Perhaps the possible "cure" that I placed my greatest hopes in was Chinese herbs. Western medicine certainly didn't have any answers. (On that topic, I can well imagine the frustration physicians must feel when confronted with a case of ALS. There is no known cause nor treatment nor, most importantly, cure.) Moreover, Chinese medicine has worked for centuries. In any event, twice a day Judy and I brewed an awful-looking concoction of a dozen or so dried "things" we had gotten at a pharmacy in Chinatown. But the looks of the brew didn't hold a candle to the horrible smell. And, unfortunately for me, the gross smell paled in comparison to the taste. Talk about foul! I dutifully drank two mugs of this broth every day for several months.

These and other hoped-for remedies — including Chinese acupressure which at least felt good — were to no avail. I am glad I tried them, however. I would have regretted not exhausting every seeming possibility.

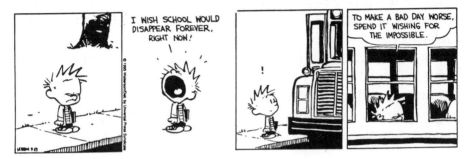

Calvin and Hobbes. Watterson. Dist. by Universal Press Syndicate.

Physical Decline

Meanwhile, my physical condition began to deteriorate more rapidly. For the first year and a couple of months my struggle was almost entirely psychological. The only physical symptoms I had were a slight weakness in my left arm and a slight limp in my left leg due to the onset of "foot drop." (This is where the muscles in the front of the leg atrophy faster than those in the back causing the front of the foot to be pulled downward. It is not painful — not until, that is, it becomes so pronounced that it causes you to trip and fall.) In fact, some neurologists thought I might have a mild case. In just over a year, from autumn 1989, through the end of 1990, however, I went from those symptoms to almost total paralysis coupled with great difficulty eating, speaking, and even breathing.

It began with my legs. I started stumbling, tripping, losing my balance. I had some harrowing falls, including one into, and through, a shower door. I progressed through a number of assistive devices for mobility: a brace to try to improve the foot drop, a regular cane to a multi-pronged one to a walker, an ordinary wheelchair to a fancy one, and two terrific battery-powered vehicles, a scooter which was perfect for school and soccer fields and an upholstered chair, called a Foxy, which was absolutely wonderful for use at home.

My other means of transportation were changing, too. I soon had to stop commuting to the university on my bike. That was a sad day because I had been enjoying that for almost 20 years. I also had to give up hiking up the eight floors to my office in favor of the elevator, a major concession. My withering left arm forced me to trade in my stick shift car for an automatic. That didn't last very long before I thought myself a menace on the road and had to depend on others to drive me to school and elsewhere.

The other difficulties I was experiencing were not so easily compensated for. My increasingly labored breathing weakened my voice making talking and especially lecturing quite a chore. Finally, due to my growing inability to swallow, I was having a hard time eating. In less than a year, I went from 170 pounds, give or take a pepperoni and extra cheese pizza, to 112. Foods I loved were steadily eliminated from my diet. Despite soft and mushy food I started choking more often leading to frequent calls to the paramedics and brief sojourns in hospital emergency rooms.

Eventually, by the end of February 1991, all of the above conditions, particularly swallowing and breathing, had gotten so bad that I was admitted to the hospital. There I was confronted with the biggest decision of my life: whether or not to go on a ventilator. A life or death decision.

With a Lot of Help from My Friends

I believe that God works through people. He is not some force that intervenes occasionally, in the style of "deus ex machina," in the affairs of humankind. God's presence in our world is a constant, living and ongoing one. It is there, obvious to anyone to see or hear, in the manifold expressions of love made by ordinary people (and the scarce extraordinary) every day.

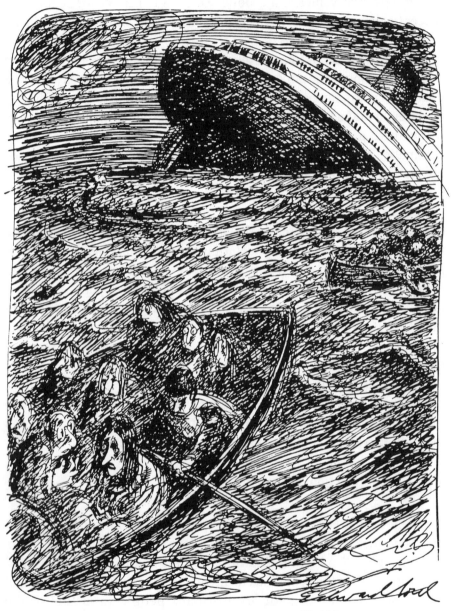

"It's probably all for the best. Those meals were awfully rich."

Drawing by Edward Sorel; ©1995 *The New Yorker Magazine*, Inc.

In the words of a beautiful song from the outstanding musical, Les Miserables, "To love another person is to see the face of God." Indeed, the gift of love, to love and be loved, is perhaps God's greatest gift. Mine is not a very complicated theology.

I did not announce my illness to anyone beyond the family and our pastor at first. By the fall of 1989, however, that something was wrong was becoming increasingly difficult to conceal from those who knew me well. (I had shrugged off questions with casual remarks that I had hurt the leg playing basketball or some such.) I remember finally telling a long-time friend, the father of one of the girls on the soccer team. He got choked up, gave me a big hug, and said, "Bob, don't ever give up."

That extremely emotional moment, simple and brief though it was, encapsulated both the great difficulty I had in telling close friends — I had trouble handling their reactions — and the immense rewards of support from doing so. Once I surmounted this very high hurdle, it seemed that everywhere my family and I looked all we could see were reflections of "the face of God." The outpouring of love and support, in words and deeds, truly astonished all of us. This blessing of love was the foundation we relied on to cope with my downhill progression.

Naturally, my most crucial source of support came from my wife, Judy, and our three children. Without their love, understanding, patience, help, humor, and enthusiasm for life, I don't know if I could have made it. Apart from specific things they did for me — including, wheelchair-bound, a marvelous visit to New York City with Judy, Laura, and our special Australian friends, Wendy and Joe O'Hara (our best buddies while in Malaysia) — they also managed to strike just the right psychological balance of sorrow and encouraging me to get on with life. That was a critical support for me.

This essential support of family is, unfortunately, not always so natural. I have heard sad stories of cases where the unafflicted spouse responded to discussion of assistive devices with a dismissive "Would that really be worth it?" It seems to me that that decision should be made by the patient. Family members who will be caregivers can have a say but the patient has the deciding vote.

Help and assistance came from all directions. Members of my extended family, both from my side as well as from Judy's, increased the frequency of their visits. They provided important physical and moral support to all of us. Our church family also came through in various ways. Pastors Dave Richardson and Maria Davis-Hanlin of Northridge United Methodist Church were invaluable sources of counsel and comfort and I talked to them often. A group of men from the church replaced the roof of our house. Others did odd jobs around the house that I could no longer do.

Friends, including ones from church and also from soccer and other areas of our lives, were equally indispensable. They inundated us with cards, notes, and prayers. Some organized to bring us delicious dinners almost every night for a number of months (until I couldn't eat much of anything). One friend, Gretchen Keeler, so persisted in her offers to be of assistance in some way or other that I overcame my ingrained reluctance to be helped and she quickly became not only my "right hand woman" but, quite literally, my right hand; as writing grew more difficult for me, she would transcribe my oral comments to written ones on student papers and exams. She also recorded the grades. (She continues to help me with various things to this day. See the chapters on "Coping.")

Another gift of love that I treasure is one from the girls on the soccer team. At the initiative of two of the moms, each of the girls contributed a personalized square for a quilt. The result was not only useful but spectacular! And very sentimental, reminding me of all the great times we had together. I was overwhelmed and I'm afraid that my thank-you speech was not too articulate.

My university also made a number of highly significant contributions. As you may know, a state university is a sizable bureaucracy within a larger bureaucracy, the university system, within the enormous bureaucracy of the state. Those bureaucracies had always been good to me but there was no reason to expect flexibility in an unusual case. Being flexible and sensitive to an individual's special needs in situations out of "the mainstream" are not, to say the least, strong suits of any bureaucracy. Yet, I was just such an unusual case. Because I loved it, I wanted to go on teaching for as long as I was able. It became clear, however, that I would need help in order to continue at all.

First, I needed to have access to the computer. My weakened arms and hands made normal use impossible. I tried a number of assistive devices but none worked adequately. Then we went to the university's Disabled Student Services and — one more blessing! We were introduced to a recent graduate who volunteered his time to work on adaptive computer devices. He designed a program that restored my ability to use the computer, via a sensor in a headband that I could trigger with my eyebrows. Some measure of independence again! More on him and his creation later.

I also needed help getting to and from campus. I was extremely fortunate to have two loyal and caring students, Steve Hirsch and Ram Srinivasan, who readily volunteered. They came to the house every morning, got me into the car, collapsed my scooter into the trunk and drove to the university where they reversed the process. At the end of the day, they repeated the whole thing and often took me to soccer games or practices. The department somehow, miraculously, found extra student assistant funds with which to pay them (though probably not for all the hours they put in). Steve and Ram became part of our family.

They and several other students with whom I was close also organized a "roast" for me in the spring of 1990. It was an extraordinary event! The large banquet room of a very nice restaurant in nearby Calabasas was packed with friends of ours — friends from all areas of our lives, soccer, church, faculty and staff from the university, girls from the soccer team, the O'Haras from Australia, and many, many of my students. To say that I was extremely flattered and honored, while true, would be a gross understatement. Overwhelmed might be more appropriate. The evening was a whole lot of fun, too. Good-natured barbs flew back and forth, I received some questionable gifts and even Mikhail Gorbachev (an impersonator who bore an uncanny resemblance to the man in the Kremlin) showed up. Yes, overwhelmed is definitely the right word for my feelings that night.

The Political Science department worked further wonders on my behalf. One of the effects of ALS is to rob you of your energy and stamina.

I had always found that teaching required a great deal of both, especially given my style of teaching compounded by having to teach the heavy load of four courses every semester. For the fall 1989 semester, after considerable internal debate because I hated to leave the classroom, I bowed to reality and accepted the kind energy-saving offer of the department chairperson, Jane Bayes, to reduce my teaching load by one course in exchange for serving as the Academic Advisor in the Dean's office. Somewhat to my surprise, I thoroughly enjoyed my three semesters in that job and, although it kept me busy, it was much less tiring than teaching and therefore helped conserve energy for my three remaining courses.

For the academic year 1990-91, my last, the department reduced my responsibilities by one more course. I kept the Model UN seminar and a lecture course on the Soviet Union. When straight lecturing became so difficult as to be impossible, the department brought in a part-timer — a young Russian woman who was a graduate student in political science at UCLA — with whom I could team-teach. She was excellent and we worked together very well.

I learned the valuable lesson that even bureaucracies can be flexible and compassionate. Like everything else, it all depends on the people involved. This goes back to what I was saying at the beginning of this section: God does indeed work through people. Ordinary people like you and me. I know this for a certainty because, in the people mentioned here and in countless others, I have seen the face of God, felt His presence, and been touched by His love. Family and friends got me through this unwelcome transition (and still sustain me). Thank you.

Without these folks, there wouldn't be any more chapters to my story. It's as simple as that.

4

THIS IS THE GOOD NEWS?

Early one morning in the hospital I woke up, feeling drugged, with a huge something in my mouth and down my throat. At least it felt enormous. And it was quite uncomfortable. A wide tube ran from the "thing" to a large, very noisy machine on a table beside my bed. In my grogginess, I also realized that I was in a different room and that I was hooked to an IV which was dripping a clear liquid into me.

I didn't remember a single bit of this happening. I tried to recall the events that had led to my current and bizarre situation. As I thought back, last evening slowly emerged from the mists of my mind. It had started out as unpleasant, gotten increasingly more difficult, and then had quickly escalated into a life-threatening crisis. The emergency situation was caused by the same problems that had brought me to the hospital in the first place, choking and difficulty breathing. I had always pulled out of these episodes with moderate help, usually a few minutes of oxygen, from paramedics and emergency room personnel (two groups for which I have the utmost respect). But not this time.

"We'll have to intubate him," I heard a doctor say when I was semiconscious and a Code Blue. And this is what they did, inserting a breathing tube down my throat. The tube was connected to a ventilator which rhythmically pumped air into and out of my lungs. This machine, with its multitude of settings and dials, requires close monitoring and that is only available in an intensive care unit where there is one nurse for every two patients. So I was in ICU.

The Decision

Intubation is only a temporary answer to breathing problems, however. Many patients are on such life support for just a short time until they no longer need it. Unfortunately, for ALS patients this is not the case. Due to the progressive weakening of the muscles, once a person goes "on the vent," it is permanent. This meant that I was still faced with the decision of whether to have a tracheotomy and be attached to a ventilator for the rest of my life, however long that might be, or not to do anything and live probably for only a short time.

It should be noted in this context that the average life expectancy of ALS patients is three to five years. I had already had the disease for two years and nine months.

It would make good reading to recount the drama of my decision-making process. I could describe my soul-searching, the agonizing discussions with physicians and clergy, tearful meditations with my family, the careful weighing of pros and cons, my intense inner struggle. These would all be normal. Perhaps it is abnormal not to have gone through these personal battles. In any case, I didn't. For me, the decision was a slam dunk, a no-brainer, a done deal, a fait accompli. So no gripping and suspenseful reading here.

I remember telling Judy, shortly after I was admitted to the hospital, that "I don't want to leave here without being able to breathe and eat more easily." That would mean a tracheotomy, with the attached ventilator, and a gastrointestinal tube. If those were what it would take, okay do it! My mind was made up. I think this was partly due to the relative suddenness with which the decision was thrust upon me. Apparently, I had naively thought that the choking and breathing problems could continue indefinitely on some sort of plateau. The error in this reasoning was that I hadn't yet reached a plateau in the progression of the disease. I really had not given the decision that much thought beforehand. My guess is that this was because, deep in my subconscious, I simply knew that I wanted to live. Period.

I certainly do not mean to minimize the significance of the decision of whether or not to go on life support. Far from it. It is obviously a monumental decision. Life on a ventilator is not easy and is often difficult and unpleasant. Your dependency on other people escalates exponentially. Moreover, a doctor confirmed my suspicion that the decision to go off the ventilator is much more difficult than deciding whether or not to go on it in the first place. Some ALS victims who have written of their experiences also warn of, and denounce, the artificiality of life on a ventilator.

For me, the pros of living so overwhelmed the cons of having to do so permanently hooked to a ventilator that it was absolutely no contest. My dependence was already total. I was paralyzed, could barely speak above a whisper, and was having greater problems eating and even breathing. What did I have to lose? I might even gain! If life on a ventilator became intolerable, well, I would cross that bridge when I came to it. As for artificiality, that sounded to me like hogwash. Sure, I would be kept alive artificially by a ventilator but my life would be real, not artificial. Or so I hoped.

This brings me to the question that is the title of this chapter: This is the good news? You already know my answer. Despite being flat on my back, largely inert, sporting fresh holes in my neck and stomach from which tubes emerged and being attached to a machine of blinking lights and luminous dials, I felt relieved and happy. I could breathe! I could eat! Well, sort of eat. At least I wouldn't be choking any more. Maybe no more urgent calls to the paramedics. And just maybe I could gain back some of the weight I had lost. A whole new world of possibilities!

In short, as I told Dave, our pastor, I felt "re-born." I didn't mean this in a particularly religious way, although faith played, and plays, a major role. I believed that I had been close to dying, and had been rescued and given a new life. I was delighted to be alive.

So, What Now?

Good question. I had absolutely no idea what lay ahead for me. Not the foggiest. I had made it through the downhill. But, through to what? I had made my decision and chosen life. What kind of life would it be? More good questions.

5

COPING I: AMAZING TECHNOLOGY

Many people have asked me how I manage to cope with my vastly altered circumstances. My fundamental answer is, "You just do." One just does. Everybody, at one time or another, is confronted with difficult situations which they didn't choose but have to work through. There is usually no "magic bullet," indeed no magic at all. This is certainly the case with me. Like a recovering alcoholic, I take one day at a time. And some days, and some weeks, are a whole lot better than others. I don't possess any great secret nor a remarkable degree of inner strength or courage. So, how do I cope? Like everyone else, I just do.

I realize this answer to the "cope question" is hardly insightful, informative, or helpful. It is inadequate. It is the truth but not the whole truth. There are, in fact, a number of specific factors that have enabled me to deal, or deal more successfully, with my new situation. Most of these have involved either amazing technology or amazing people, often both. The support has been there in several forms and I have sought to take advantage of it all.

Getting My Act Together

I had to develop some new traits and strengthen some existing ones in order to have any hope of coping. Far and away, the most important was one that had never been among my stronger attributes: patience. This was not easily done but was essential. There is simply no option, other than driving yourself and everyone around you crazy, for a person who is paralyzed and on a ventilator. I was completely helpless and completely dependent. Learning patience has been a lengthy process for me; suffice to say, I still have room for improvement but I have come a long way.

Speaking of patience, I began to run out of it after three weeks in the hospital. I had adapted to the ventilator and grown accustomed to my food, Osmolite HN. I had stopped losing weight and had regained some degree of energy. It was all very encouraging and I was ready to go home. (Besides, the hospital didn't have cable TV and I was missing some good programs, particularly on CNN, A&E, and ESPN. The hospital did have a channel on which it showed videos in the evenings; one nurse even brought in a few from his own collection that he thought I might enjoy. I did.) Despite my escalating bugging of my doctors, I was destined for another week in ICU. This time was necessary to finish weaning me off various pain-killers and for me to adjust to the smaller, portable ventilator I would be using at home.

We did a couple of intelligent things while I was in the hospital. One was obvious: we hung my communication board from an empty arm of the IV or, later when I was off IVs, feeding pole. This enabled me to express my needs and even some thoughts to medical personnel, at least those who had the patience to spell with me (which most had). I could also communicate with visitors.

Actually, the name "communication board" perhaps implies that it was more sophisticated than it really was. It was a very simple alphabet chart that my disappearing voice forced my helper, Gretchen, and me to create during one afternoon of grading. It has five rows of letters, a through e, f through j, and so on; the speaking person then only had to say the numbers 1 through 5 and then the letters in the line which I indicated by raising my eyebrows. Since then, I have become aware of more sophisticated devices — from charts with the alphabet arranged by frequency of use (like my computer program) to a see-through piece of plastic with the letters grouped in quadrants and where the speaker can see where you are looking. Nevertheless, we have stuck with our original "no-frills" version, adding only two rows of numbers. It seems to me that this basic means of communication has the advantages of being convenient and easy to use for novices as well as a tool for reasonably rapid conversation for experienced users.

(Such alphabet charts are a cumbersome means of communicating basic and regular needs, however. The answer is a separate chart which somehow lists those needs. Judy made a large chart for the wall of my bedroom as soon as I got home from the hospital. It has "a" through "g" along the top and "1" through "9" down the side. The resulting 63 spaces were remarkably easy to fill, with items including Food, Juice, Suction, Change TV Channel, Urinal, Alphabet Chart, Get Judy, Move Head, Turn Me, and so on.)

The second smart move was not as obvious; in fact, we did it only at the suggestion of my physician brother-in-law, Kim. After making sure it would be okay with the nurses, we took our newly hired caregiver to the hospital with me. Mario had been with us for only a few weeks, part-time, but he seemed very capable — especially in light of his first evening of work when he handled a choking episode, the paramedics and the emergency room well and unflappably. He was there for four hours a day and the nurses trained him in everything, from settings on the ventilator, feeding and bathing me, to the art of suctioning. This training has proved invaluable; Mario soon became full-time and is now my main caregiver.

Upon arriving home, I quickly disabused myself of two personal illusions. The first to go was the belief that I had regained much of my energy. In reality, I was pooped! For the first two months or so, I rested a great deal and watched an inordinate amount of television. The second illusion that I shed concerned food. I had fervently hoped to be able to eat such things as soup, mashed potatoes, and ice cream. I craved them, almost an obsession. The doctors had been noncommittal so one night I tried some very creamy mashed potatoes with gravy. Big mistake. They tasted great but "went down the wrong way" and we were suctioning them for the next week. I learned and have had no "real" food since that one experiment.

When I wasn't watching television, I did undertake one "active" and constructive project. Since I still felt like a teacher and still received a number of academic journals, I read. I tried to keep current in my fields of specialization. Nearly every morning, after reading the newspaper and the previous day's mail — and, of course, checking the TV schedule — I would spend anywhere from half an hour to almost two hours reading a variety of journals that the nurse propped on my lap desk.

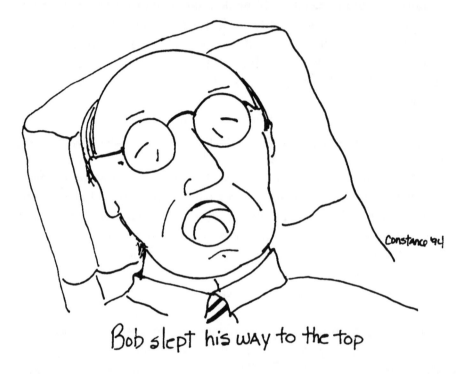

Bob slept his way to the top

Contoons by Constance Houck

In retrospect, I think this simple activity played a major role in my ability to cope with my illness. This has been true all throughout my struggle with the disease, but especially in the first few months following my release from the hospital. It represented a connection to normalcy, to something that I was used to doing. Moreover, reading my academic journals also gave me an interest beyond myself. Both of these were of critical importance in helping me not to dwell on my helpless condition but rather to focus on something that I could do and that stimulated my mind.

As I gradually gained increased degrees of energy and stamina, I found that I needed more outlets. This is where technology comes in.

"Practical" Technology

The advances made in assistive devices of all kinds over the years, especially recently, has provided new opportunities and greater independence to people with disabilities. I am able to do a range of things that a person like me could not have done less than a generation ago.

Technology for medical-related equipment has been of particular assistance in facilitating my mobility. For example, after I got home from the hospital, I could be moved out to my reclining chair — which is far more comfortable than any wheelchair my fanny had ever been plopped into — in the living room by any two people lifting me from my adjustable hospital bed into the wheelchair, pushing me the short distance between rooms and then lifting me from the wheelchair into my recliner. Except for negotiating a couple of very tight turns, it was not a difficult process. However, as I began to regain weight, lifting me did start to become a problem and I would often find myself perched precariously between the wheelchair and the bed or the chair. It was time — past time from my point of view and way past time from that of my lifters', especially Judy's — to find a new mode of transporting me.

We had previously experimented with a Trans Aid version of a Hoyer lift. I hadn't particularly enjoyed being suspended in the air by a net sling and four lengths of chains. Now, however, there didn't seem to be any choice. I eventually got used to it — but I still don't find it comfortable — and it has proved to be enormously convenient. Now, it only takes one person to move me and, true to its name, the lift does all the lifting. (I bypass the wheelchair and am rolled in the lift directly from the bed to the chair and back again.)

Wheelchairs vary greatly. My current wheelchair is a much more sophisticated contraption than the standard, basic model I had earlier. The back adjusts to any angle from almost straight upright to nearly flat. The legs or feet do the same. The arm rests are relatively soft molded plastic and also are adjustable. Since I have no neck muscles, the headrest is a must. Finally, it has room underneath for both a ventilator and an attached battery.

My ventilator is a true marvel of modern technology. It measures an incredibly compact 8½ inches high by 12½ wide by just 11½ deep. I continue to be amazed that such a relatively tiny machine is breathing for me and keeping me alive. After the first month when we had some trouble due to the wrong tubing and a couple of less than competent nurses, both the main vent and the back-up have been extremely reliable. (No matter how dependable a machine may be, a back-up is absolutely essential. This is true for ventilators as well as suction machines, portable suction machines, and batteries.) Almost as importantly, it is so portable that anyone can lift it and it fits conveniently on a shelf Mario built for the lift, both of which gives me mobility at home; and it fits just as smoothly on the tray under my wheelchair, which gives me great mobility on the "outside."

"Recreational" Technology

There are three key "recreational" technological items which have immeasurably aided my ability to cope: a van, a page turner and a computer. All expanded my independence and freedom. They have been invaluable.

A van with a wheelchair lift is virtually a necessity. The problem is, however, that they are quite expensive. We have been very fortunate in this regard as we have enjoyed the luxury of a free "loaner." Our good friends, Lew and Joyce Herbst, have loaned us their van for as long as I need it — after making it accessible by removing all but two seats and having a lift and wheelchair moorings installed. It has been terrific!

The van has given me the freedom to go anywhere within a reasonable driving distance. One and a half to two hours seems to be my maximum but I prefer somewhat shorter trips. The preparation and the journey itself are tiring for me and I want to have energy left to enjoy my destination. I suppose I go somewhere in the van once a week on average; due to the hassle and the fact that I have a lot of things I enjoy doing at home, that is enough for me.

One hour's drive from our home in the San Fernando Valley in any direction gets you to a huge number of Los Angeles area attractions. These include the beach, mountains and desert as well as museums, theaters, and sports venues. Most of my early trips (other than to doctors' appointments), however, were to none of these. They were to church, less than 10 minutes from our house, for Sunday morning worship services. I had hoped, quite unrealistically as I soon discovered, to be there for that first post-hospital Easter but I was still too weak in April to venture out. I finally made it to my first service while on the ventilator in November and I will never forget the thrill of that long-awaited day. Not only did it mark my "coming out," as it were, but it was also the very first service in our new sanctuary. Finally being present at a worship service, in our beautiful new church, and seeing so many of our friends was wonderful and also extremely emotional. Getting to church, for worship services and music programs, has continued to be a high priority for us. And we haven't missed an Easter Sunday service since that first year.

Incidentally, Judy has become quite adept at getting me, single-handedly, to church and on other outings. The lift makes it possible for one person to move me from the bed to the wheelchair. The tricky parts are positioning me properly in the wheelchair and the return trip to bed when the sling from the lift and I have moved — in different directions. Once I am set in the wheelchair, a velcro strap is used to secure my head. With my head unable to flop forward or slip sideways, I can ride in the van without an additional attendant. This is not ideal, especially on freeway jaunts, and the whole process is tiring for Judy, but it has greatly enhanced our flexibility and independence.

I extended and increased my forays into the outside world only very, very gradually. My enforced idleness naturally escalated my love for listening to classical music, especially Mozart, as well as jazz, country, older rock and roll ("Oldies But Goodies"), and certain other kinds of music; this necessitated periodic visits to the local CD emporium to augment my collection. My love of reading led to similar trips to a bookstore. I made it to several girls' soccer games. Eventually, I got up the nerve to try a museum and our tour of an exhibit on Catherine the Great worked out quite well. Another trip was to the beach at Channel Islands Harbor, near Oxnard, to see friends. This journey also went smoothly, except for one tiny problem.

All mechanical devices are subject to breakdowns, of course. Our van and its lift have been no exception. The lift's problem was frustrating in the extreme. It would work fine one day or one trip or one way and then on the next get stuck before completely lowering or raising (often with me on it). We took it to the mechanics who had installed the lift, repeatedly, and they would either do nothing and tell us it was fine or charge us the proverbial arm and leg for something that had no effect whatever on the glitch. Finally, a friend figured out the problem and fixed it, at a cost of $12 for the part and it's been working perfectly, knock on wood, ever since. Before the Case of the Temperamental Lift was solved, however, the problem aborted several trips, usually on arrival, and/or necessitated manually lifting me into or out of the van.

Most people, I suppose, have experienced a vehicle breakdown while on the road. But how many of those have been with a disabled person in the car or van, especially one confined to a wheelchair? Such events vary from minor inconveniences to near-crises. An example of the former was the time the van quit on the way home from church. We were only a little over a mile from the house, so we walked. Or, more accurately, I rode while Judy and my nurse du jour took turns pushing.

We were not so lucky the next time, though. This was the occasion of the "tiny problem" I mentioned. It was Sunday of a Memorial Day weekend and we had enjoyed a great trip to the beach and visit with friends. When the van conked out on the steep Camarillo grade on the way home, however, our adventure was just beginning. It was easy to know what to do about the van but what to do about moi ? I couldn't very well be hoisted up into the cab of the tow truck. Angel, our nurse, then hit on the obvious, and seemingly only, solution: an ambulance. For the next two and a half hours we pursued that answer only to be stymied at every turn. The responses to our plight included: we can only take you to a hospital, only to the nearest hospital, and (my personal favorite) we can't cross county lines. We tried other alternatives with the same results. The only offer we had was to take us home for a mere $553. Right!

During this increasingly frustrating ordeal we did have one thing going for us: a guardian angel in the form of Tammy, a CHP officer. She stayed with us the entire time providing invaluable moral support. She also handled most of our phone calls and even came up with the means of getting us home. She spotted an airport shuttle with wheelchair access and persuaded the company to pick us up. The shuttle company went out of their way, too, as legally they are only supposed to go between home and airport. We shall always remain grateful to Tammy and the shuttle.

To me, this saga was a morality play. It was about the struggle between the dark forces of bureaucracy and the forces of light, humanity. Humanity eventually triumphed. That is one moral of this tale. Another is that we should have been in church. It would have been a whole lot simpler.

The van's successes have vastly outnumbered its failures. Nevertheless, I am glad that I don't have to go out to be satisfied. As much as I enjoy the outdoors, I am content to be at home most of the time. This is because I love to read and to write. Technology has made both of these feasible and doable. On the reading front, I have an electric page turner which has been terrific. When I began to have real difficulty holding a book, much less turning pages, we started to scout around for some device that would do those for me. After all, reading was a major part of my profession and I had been doing it all my life. I couldn't just give it up; at least I didn't want to, not without a fight.

There are a plethora of such gadgets on the market, ranging from the very basic to the quite sophisticated. Prices vary accordingly. Since Judy and I were ignorant in such matters, we asked my knowledgeable physical therapist if she had any advice. She did and, naturally, she recommended the most expensive one. Not really. What she did was recommend a page turner that would "grow with me," that is, compensate for the progression of the disease. It just happened that it was also near the top end of the price scale. But it was invaluable advice. The machine I have — a "Gewa" which, I was told, was made in Sweden and is obtainable from Zygo Industries in Portland, Oregon — has indeed evolved with my physical deterioration. When I got it, I still had muscles in my neck so I could operate it by touching a lever with my chin. After these muscles gave out, however, such "chinning" was no longer possible. No problem! With the attachment of a scanning device, I was able to read at least as easily as before. When the scanner lights up the movement I want — move the roller forward or backward and turn the page forward or backward — I trigger the machine into action via a sensor hooked to a signal switch box. In turn, I trigger the sensor either by raising my eyebrows against a headband or by nudging a foot pedal. Piece of cake! Well, almost.

There have been problems. One of the cables unexpectedly wears out, or the sensor does. The battery in the box runs down. The headband is too tight or too loose. The sensor was in the wrong spot on my forehead. It was often difficult to find the source of the problem. Sometimes the problem was me, if, for instance, I was tired and not raising my eyebrows effectively. In fact, eventually my eyebrows weakened to the point that I had to abandon the headband in favor of the foot pedal. It is not quite as convenient and it's slower but at least I can work it.

By whatever means I operate it, my page turner has been a godsend. After it is set up, I am completely independent (except when some pages stick together which they occasionally do), not having to rely on anyone. Such independence is extremely rare for people in my situation and I greatly treasure it. Moreover, a good book can be a refreshing and perspective-restoring momentary escape from my problems. Since I am confronted with my physical limitations every minute of every day, these diversions are as invaluable as my periods of independence.

After emerging from the hospital at the end of March 1991, with some tubes and a ventilator, I spent the next couple of months recuperating and regaining some measure of energy. I didn't do much during those months. What ultimately spurred me into "action" was a gift from a close friend and colleague of a novel by one of my favorite British authors. I was anxious to read it and that meant trying out the new accessories to the page turner, the scanner, and the headband. I was somewhat surprised to discover that they worked, or, rather, that I was able to work them. I loved the book and went on to read almost 50 more books via the page turner by the end of the year. Over the following three years, I devoured almost 300 additional books with the help of that wonderful machine.

All kinds of books — on Russia and the Soviet Union, on Asia, on current events, histories, biographies, and novels of all sorts. I am thoroughly enjoying the opportunity to do mostly "recreational" reading which there was never time for when I was teaching.

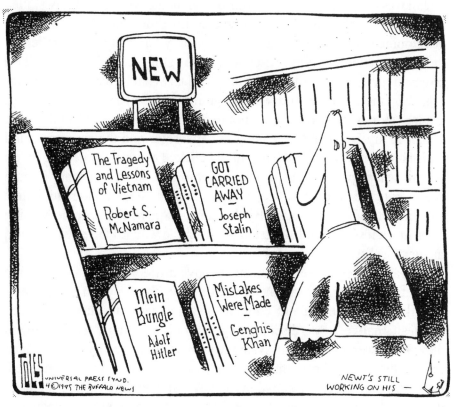

For writing, I needed a computer with a special program and a means of accessing it. I already had a computer, a Macintosh, on which I had done course syllabi, lecture notes, simulation materials, research notes, articles, and papers for several years. I knew the machine, liked it, and preferred to keep using it if at all possible. My arms had grown too weak to lift to the keyboard, however, and a trip through the Disabled Student

Services lab at the university revealed no immediately appealing alternative. Then Gail Pickering, a very knowledgeable and patient specialist at the center, came up with the key idea of introducing us to a young man by the name of Jan Motil.

Jan was a recent Cal State Northridge graduate who was highly skilled in computer technology. He volunteered his time and talents at the lab developing computer programs for physically handicapped members of the university community. After hearing my story, he offered to design a program for me that could be run on my Mac. What he came up with was a grid of the alphabet and various grammatical marks down which a scanner slowly moved; when it got to the line I wanted, I would click a sensor in my headband by raising my eyebrows and the scanner would cruise horizontally along the line until I clicked again at the desired letter. It was a slow process but, at the same time, a wonderful one. I could again write notes for my classes, comments on books I had read, letters and all sorts of other things. (By this time, I was having trouble holding a pen much less accomplishing anything legible with it.) Jan's work served me very well for three years.

By early 1993, however, I began to have difficulty using the program due mainly, I think, to marginally weakened eyebrows. Two friends, who were knowledgeable about computers, volunteered to launch a search for an alternative. It was discouraging. The only seemingly feasible option they found was an elaborate system which one operated by looking at an area on the screen. From the brochure I studied and the video I watched, it was an extremely attractive system. What was unattractive about it, though, was its price tag of over $20,000. It was just too expensive, especially considering that, with ALS, my longevity was in doubt. I decided against it.

We then hit on the idea of calling our friend Gail Pickering at the university. We should have called her right in the beginning because she had an excellent recommendation. On a Friday afternoon, about a week later, Diane Bristow, a specialist in adaptive computer devices, came to our house with a bag full of goodies. What excited me were two programs she had on her PowerBook. One was a word processing program, Microsoft Word, and the other was a word prediction program called

Co:Writer. The latter could be a real time-saver because it gives you four possibilities for your word every time you typed a letter; when the word you wanted showed up on the list, all you had to do was type its number, 1 through 4. Not only would this be faster than my existing program, but the combination would also "reunite" me with familiar and valuable word processing functions such as editing and saving. Both programs work by scanning grids and the two mesh together beautifully.

It sounded too good to be true. And, unfortunately, it was. For me, the flaw was in how the program was operated. I just couldn't blink or move my eyes at the right time to trigger the infrared sensor, attached to my glasses, when the scanner arrived at the line or letter I wanted. Diane left the entire setup with us for the weekend so that I could practice. To no avail. Moreover, I found it extremely fatiguing. Judy did, too, and was no more successful than I was. After 20 minutes of concentrated effort, my brother, Tom, had typed "dog" and had a raging headache. I was very disappointed when we had to tell Diane that it was a "no go" when she and Gail came over to pick it up that Monday. It had looked so promising.

This story has a happy ending, however. During our conversation with Diane and Gail, I got Judy's attention like I normally do when we are not making eye contact, by raising my foot the quarter of an inch or so that I can lift it. (Among the very few muscles I have left are limited lifting ones in my thighs.) They looked surprised, if not shocked, and one of them asked me if I could do it voluntarily. I raised my eyebrows in the affirmative and demonstrated a few of my "leg kicks" for them. With a laughing "Well, why didn't you say so?" Diane dipped into her bag of tricks and extracted an odd-looking object. It had a clamp on one end and a "rocking" switch mounted on the other, with several adjustable bends and extensions in between. To my utter amazement, when the clamp was attached to the foot of my halfway reclined chair, I could operate the switch by raising my foot and, thus, OPERATE THE COMPUTER AND ITS PROGRAMS!!! Needless to say, I was thrilled. Now, I could use these wonderful programs.

Diane gave us specific recommendations for the software and the hardware. When the programs and the new, larger computer arrived, she came over and installed and set up everything. It seemed, at a cost of about $3,500, to be an investment worth the risk. That it has been indeed! Since June 1993, I have accomplished what seems to me to be an extraordinary amount and have saved much of it on the hard disk to prove it. And I have loved it.

Of course, using my foot is not as fast as using my hands. But, then, my hands are not available. And my foot is not all that slow. Besides, as a friend pointed out to me, using my feet rather than my hands is quite appropriate for an old soccer coach. A common soccer slogan found on tee shirts and other paraphernalia is "Soccer is for kicks." Well, trust me, computers are, too!

I marvel at all these technological innovations and how they have improved and enriched my life. They have increased my independence and enabled me to challenge my physical limitations. Technology doesn't exist in a vacuum, however. There have been key people involved in every one of these technological benefits.

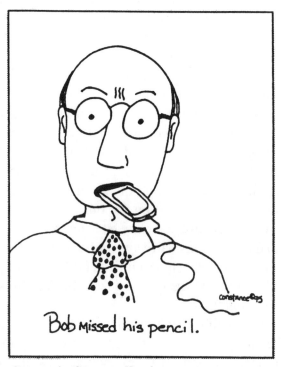

Contoons by Constance Houck

6

Coping II: Wondrous People

My story is really just as much about other people as it is about me. Technological advances have made my life more productive and fulfilling than many, including this writer, would have thought possible. It is people, however, who give meaning to life and make it worth living. It is people who you encounter along the way who provide life with its vibrant colors and rich textures.

I have been extremely fortunate in the "people department." When I was "normal," I was surrounded by a diverse group of good, interesting, and fun people. And ever since I began my "descent into abnormality" with the onset of ALS, most of that large group has remained steadfast in its support. Moreover, it has even grown! I have heard from friends that I hadn't been in touch with for years. Casual friends from soccer and church have gone out of their way for us.

One of the most common, and poignant, complaints among ALS victims — and perhaps others with severe disabilities or terminal illnesses — is how some friends just disappear when the going get tough. I can't say that I haven't experienced this painful phenomenon. And I can't pretend that it doesn't hurt. I have seen several friends drop out of my life and the hurt has been deep. I am not entirely sure why these particular people have drifted away. Maybe some of them were not such good friends after all. More likely, I think, is that many of them, perhaps the vast majority, just can't deal with my disease. This may be because they can't stand to see a friend reduced to my condition or because I am a reminder of their own mortality or a combination of both. In any case, I prefer not to criticize those relative few but rather to applaud the many who have been of such help to me.

Simply put, living with this disease is difficult in any case but I would dread having to face it with no outside support. I don't think it would be possible. Not to be melodramatic, but loving, caring people make a critical difference, the difference between life and death.

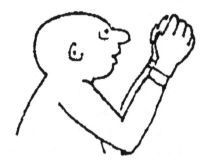

Dear God, let me tell you how I want this prayer answered!

Cartoon by David Richardson

Hurdles and Hurdlers

What most amazes me is that whenever I reached a turning point in the progression of the disease, someone would suddenly appear with a solution. God does indeed work in mysterious ways sometimes. The more I think about it, though, the more the ways don't seem so mysterious because they have been so consistent. Shortly after a problem would pop up, a person or a group of them with an answer would, too.

I have already introduced most of these people. My family, immediate and extended, has risen to the occasion right from the beginning with understanding, encouragement and, as always, a healthy dose of humor.

When I needed someone to talk things through with, I could always count on Dave Richardson and often my peripatetic brother, Tom. Colleagues at the university were sensitive to my need to lighten my teaching load. When I needed help getting to and from school, students of mine volunteered their assistance. And, when hauling me in and out of a normal car became too awkward and I was pretty much confined to a wheelchair, Lew and Joyce Herbst offered to have their van converted to make it accessible for my use.

The Keelers also deserve to be near the top of this list of various people coming to my aid at different times and in a variety of ways. Gretchen still comes over faithfully every other week to help me with things I can't do myself. She has become my "official" research assistant for this book; among other duties, she keeps my notes organized, provides useful and necessary feedback on what I have written, and makes frequent library runs. To be fair, I increased her salary substantially, from zero to double that amount. Her husband, Bruce, recently volunteered to help me with the Slugs, my fantasy baseball team. His offer came at a critical time because Judy was rebelling against having to do it. Bruce has already been of major assistance, we are working together very well (communicating by fax) and, most important, we are both enjoying it greatly. And, since my bankroll was depleted by the sizable raise I gave Gretchen, I gave Bruce a new title. He is the new, and first ever, Director of Player Personnel. I remain owner, and drumroll please, Boss.

Two prominent examples of the right people appearing unexpectedly on my horizon at the right time were my "computer gurus," Jan and Diane (and I owe much thanks to Gail who introduced me to both of them). They were, are, exceptional. I hate to think of how many hours Jan must have put in on my behalf. He was never satisfied and was constantly working to improve his original creation. Every time he came up with a new version, he would spend a whole evening with me in my study having me test it and make suggestions. Then he would go home and work on it some more. We finally settled on version six or seven! His dedication, especially for someone who was volunteering his time, was just outstanding.

I wrote a letter to Diane a month or two after I was "up and running" on the new system that she had recommended and then installed. Here is what I said to her:

> I sing your praises — to myself, needless to say, but sung nevertheless — every time I use this new computer and its programs. And I use it almost every day. I am loving it!
>
> Just why, you ask? Let me count the ways. I love the independence, that I can "do it all" once it is turned on and the foot switch properly positioned. I am greatly enjoying the word processing; I again have all the flexibility to edit, format, save, and so on that I used to have. The word prediction is terrific (and sometimes quite funny) and saves all kinds of time. I also appreciate the bigger and color monitor. Enough said?
>
> I hold you personally responsible for all of this. And I am extremely grateful. Thank you for your expertise, your patience in exploring the various options, your observation of my slight foot movement, and your skill in installing all the programs and setting up the whole thing. Without you, we would not have even known about this adaptive equipment and, of course, we wouldn't have had a prayer of setting it up.
>
> The end result is that I don't get nearly as tired as I used to with my old program with the headband. Combined with all the other advantages means that writing is fun again.
>
> Many, many thanks.

There are also some people that I haven't introduced, at least not in this context. One of the major burdens the family of an ALS victim faces in financial. Sooner, rather than later, most patients are going to require some level of nursing care. How much depends on the amount of responsibility the spouse, if there is one, is willing and able to assume. How skilled depends on the stage of the disease. Before I went on the ventilator, I need only part-time, relatively unskilled help; once hooked to the ventilator, however, I required around-the-clock skilled care. This is extraordinarily expensive, as you can imagine, even if insurance picks up part of the tab. Moreover, this financial burden comes at a time when the family income has usually been slashed by the patient's disability. (It should be noted that ALS strikes a disproportionately higher percentage of men than women.)

Seeing this financial nightmare looming imminently, a group of our friends decided to do something about it. Without our involvement, they established a fund, straightforwardly named The Bob Horn Fund, and sent a letter to a number of our friends explaining the situation and requesting contributions. The response overwhelmed me! In fact, in continues to astonish me because the fund still exists to this day. It has been of enormous assistance in defraying the high cost of my care. Judy and I are forever grateful to these kind and generous people — although we don't know who they are. The treasurer of the fund, Chloe Sidwell, acknowledges each contribution but to us they are anonymous. All we can do is offer our heartfelt thanks.

Another, albeit lesser, burden is trips to the doctor's office. Not only is it a hassle getting me ready, but there is the hassle of coordinating the schedules of the doctor, Judy, a caregiver, and me. Miraculously, my physician, Gordon Dowds, makes house calls! Yet another example of the wonder of people, hurdlers of obstacles!

Field Trips

My gradually increasing ventures out hit a peak — so far, that is — in 1994. The year began with the devastating Northridge earthquake, an inauspicious beginning to a year for greater excursions. My two-week hospitalization, starting on the morning of the quake but largely unrelated to it, and subsequent recuperation wiped out most of the next two months. But that natural disaster also was a catalyst in creating a new option in my still narrow range of outing possibilities. Since we hadn't suffered extensive damage in the earthquake, the Federal Emergency Management Agency gave us only a very small sum for immediate repairs to certain pipes and the water heater and for a chimney inspection. Part of the latter was a smoke test and the inspectors from the company we had hired required that I be out of the house for a few hours while they did that.

What to do? We finally decided to try a movie, which I had been reluctant to attempt because of the noise of the ventilator, the probable need for suctioning, and the myriad other personal and logistical details. However, the movie was loud enough, my needs were minimal, I loved seeing a film again, and I suppose we averaged a movie a month for the rest of the year. That first movie, *Schindler's List,* is, incidentally, one of the best films I have ever seen.

In the summer, my basketball buddy, Martin Turley, offered to take me on some trips. Martin had been coming over on a regular basis for several months and Judy had trained him on the ventilator, how to suction, and so on. He is a special education teacher for grades K-6 and had time in the summer. The most significant aspect of these proposed outings was that they would be the first (except for a couple of local trips with my brother Tom) without Judy; I would be in the hands of a caregiver whose English is severely limited and a "rookie." But I need not have worried. With Mario taking care of me and Martin handling logistics and serving as our tour guide, all three of our legendary trips went, as a Brit might say, "swimmingly."

Our first "field trip" was to the fascinating Gene Autry Western Heritage Museum in the Griffith Park area of Los Angeles. The second was to see two exciting and beautiful films on Africa and Hawaii on the gigantic screen of the IMAX Theater, located down on the University of Southern California campus. I considered both ventures out to be quite ambitious. But our third was even more so. We took the train, the new Metrolink, into downtown LA where we connected with the still-in-progress subway system. We rode to a park, where we had lunch, and then to the rebuilt Central Library. At the latter, we poked around and eventually located its copy of the book I had written; it was water-marked from the fire. Then it was the subway to beautiful old Union Station where we caught the train for home. It was a long but wonderful day. The weather was gorgeous, not a cloud or trace of smog, the renovated library spectacular, the subway convenient and clean, and the train trip very interesting (I love trains!). Martin and Mario enjoyed the day as much as I did.

This trip, in particular, necessitates a few remarks about accessibility. I was amazed at the provision for wheelchairs in both the train and subway: entrance to the cars was easy, there were designated places for wheelchairs and entrances to and exits from stations were made convenient by elevators. Moreover, there always seemed to be an "official" person around making sure we were all right, answering questions, and giving directions. In other trips, we have found a similar sensitivity to disabled people and greatly improved access. This access includes everything from cuts in sidewalks — in New York in 1990, however, there were a total of none on our various routes — to elevators and ramps, special seating, and the list goes on and on. This enhanced accessibility opens up a vast array of opportunities for the disabled to enjoy all kinds of "normal" activities.

Three other 1994 journeys are worth mentioning because they were extra-special. The first was nostalgic, a trip partly from the past and partly of the present, coupled with major role reversals for all involved. *Our three children took ME to Dodger Stadium for a ball game!* They were quite brave in carrying through with their Father's Day gift because, with Judy back East visiting her family, they were responsible for the whole nine yards. They pulled it off without a hitch and we had a wonderful time together — lovely evening, excellent seats, and a great game that the home team won. It was so good to be back in one of my favorite haunts again after an absence of four years.

The other two very special outings were a little way up the California coast. One was a long-awaited excursion to Santa Barbara, specifically to UCSB, to see Laura. We took her to lunch — despite the various and comparatively exotic temptations, I had the usual, an infusion of good old Osmolite — bought several items at the newly renovated campus bookstore where she worked, and visited the apartment she shared with five other girls. Then Laura took us to the women's soccer match; we won and the three girls I had coached played terrifically. A wonderful day!

The other trip was to Oxnard, this side of Santa Barbara, to the "beach house" which we owned with two other families — for an overnight! In fact, four nights, my first nights away from home (other than those spent in the hospital) in almost five years. My whole family was coming for Thanksgiving — my Mom from Detroit, my brother and his family from Pittsburgh, and my sister and her family from Juneau; eight in all — and we knew that hosting them in our house would be somewhere between uncomfortable and impossible. The beach house, on the other had, has a much larger living room, more bedrooms and bathrooms, and obviously but crucially, was at the beach. A perfect alternative! Except it meant moving me and all my *barang-barang* (the Indonesian term for baggage or, more broadly, "stuff"). The logistics were daunting. Nevertheless, with Judy organizing, my brother Tom and Mario stuffed the latter's pickup with my hospital bed and reclining chair, the lift, a small table, a backup ventilator, and two extra suction machines. Then the only remaining problem was to get my esteemed but deadweight self up the stairs to the main living area of the beach house; this was accomplished by scores of people (not really) huffing and puffing (really) to carry me up in a sheet. Thanks to everyone pitching in with help, it was a special thanksgiving, a wonderful family time and a refreshing vacation for me. I returned home tired but exhilarated.

If the remainder of 1995 keeps up with the pace of its first month, however, this year's number of trips will exceed those of 1994. We made it to church twice. I also saw my first basketball game in several years with my friend of almost 25 years Jay Lyter, who organized the excursion to UCLA, and Martin. This trip marked another first because it was without either Judy or Mario. Jay and Martin were, however, very attentive to my needs and we had a great time with no significant problems. And the eventual NCAA champion Bruins won! Finally, January produced yet another first: live theater. In fact, we saw three plays at three different theaters! Judy and I both love "the theatre" and it was wonderful to be back.

A word about "firsts." A bunch of words, actually. New adventures are just that, adventures. Your driver may not be familiar with the route or, importantly in the case of a van and for someone who has to push the wheelchair, with the parking situation. For example, the Music Center in downtown Los Angeles, where we saw *Miss Saigon,* has very convenient underground parking with a reasonable clearance of six-and-a-half feet; so, it was essential to know, *ahead of time,* that our van is a wee bit higher at 6'8". Other confusions may occur concerning access and seating, to name just two. I avoided allowing such unknowns or other apprehensions to deter me from going on these various outings. The watchwords, as for every activity of a disabled person, are: plan ahead as much as possible, allow plenty of time and, above all, be flexible and prepared to "go with the flow."

My OPB

And, now, a word from my sponsor. I get a lot of books as gifts and personally buy quite a few, either at one of the local book emporiums or by mail-order. But the bulk of the steady inflow of books come from my Official Procurer of Books. That is my Mom. I don't recall the precise circumstances surrounding the origin of this delightful arrangement. She must have offered once to purchase the books on a list I had compiled. In my naturally unassuming way, I took it as a deal in perpetuity. Mom has yet to rebel when, every three or four months, I send her a list of 12 or 14 "desperately needed" tomes. The folks at the neighborhood Walden Books rejoice when they see her coming. Evidently, they love me, too, to judge from a ditty Mom dashed off recently:

> When your list I did see,
> Away did I flee,
> To Walden's, the fountain of knowledge!
> Their eyes lit with glee
> When me they did see.
> Said Walden, "Now my kids can afford college."
> When all's done and said,
> Walden's will be out of the red
> "And we owe it all to your Robbie.
> We want you to know we do love him so,
> And we're happy he reads as a hobby."

Jay and Martin

I have already introduced these two friends who have taken me on a number of enjoyable of field trips. But they have done more, much more. When we lost our nursing coverage — see following chapter — both of them volunteered to be trained as caregivers. None of our other friends, with the exception of Dave, did and I can't say that I blame them. Not only is there a lot to learn but it is a huge responsibility. Now both put in regular stints taking care of me, enabling Judy to attend meetings or enjoy a well-deserved break. That is friendship above and beyond. If I could, and if I wore one, I would doff my hat to them!

Due to these and other friends, I have not joined one of the many available ALS support groups. They are undeniably of significant assistance to many people, but I seem to be doing quite well with my "private" support group of family and friends.

The bottom line? Technology is amazing. And people are even more so!

PART THREE

AFFIRMING LIFE

7

SHIFT CHANGE!

Short ones. Tall ones. Fat and thin, male and female, black and white and Asian, straight and gay, young and old, competent and incompetent. Representatives from at least two dozen countries and every continent except Antarctica. A diverse group, to say the least, of nurses and caregivers has paraded through my life and the house the past three years. As with everything else in life, only the last counts in nursing care. When you are dependent on a nurse, you don't care if the person is green with three heads. You only care that they are competent. None of the rest makes one whit of difference. At least, it doesn't to me.

Fortunately, I have had a number of excellent nurses and caregivers. They have been skilled, caring, observant, able to communicate, and often with an enjoyable sense of humor. Unfortunately, I have also had a succession of incompetents and/or dingbats. This chapter, then, is about them, all of them, good, bad, and indifferent. It is dedicated, with affection and appreciation, to the good ones. I owe them a great deal.

Hospital Nurses

My experience with nurses — and with respiratory therapists — during my month-long sojourn in the hospital in March 1991, was almost uniformly positive. The ICU personnel were highly skilled. Reflecting back, some were friendlier than others, some more patient, and some seemed more caring. Although I began to notice such differences in the latter part of my stay, they hardly mattered. They were inconsequential, trivial. I was, as they say, just damn glad to be there. Here. Among the living. Alive! Besides, how did I know what the nurses were doing to me, much less what should have been done, if different, or how anything should be done? I was new at all this. And I was completely clueless.

The only real problems I had with my nurses occurred twice a day, every day. At 7AM and 7PM (with minor, usually, turmoil at 3 in the afternoon and 11 in the evening) came the dreaded SHIFT CHANGE. (Eerie music, on an organ. Vincent Price in a cape, looking diabolical as only he could. The phantom of the Paris opera house in a particularly foul mood, really bummed out about something or other. That's the picture.) Everyone who has spent time in a hospital has observed this pernicious phenomenon. It is a designated period when absolutely every nurse, bar none, incoming and outgoing and even those just staying on, hides. Yep, hides. Really. Some, brazenly, have the gall to hide in plain sight!

The nurses heading home, or wherever, need this time to impart important information about their patients to the ones coming on duty. This is valuable, of course. The problem, however, is that they are all in absentia at the same time. Heaven help you if you need something during those 15 or 20 minutes. Maybe, just maybe, someone will come, reluctantly, to your aid. This very unpleasant aspect of shift changes escalates to near-panic when the patient is not able to press a call button or even shout. It forced us to try to have someone, mainly Judy or Mario, with me during all shift changes. This required some acrobatic schedule juggling, especially by Judy, but it worked well because she and Mario were able either to satisfy whatever my need was or, very occasionally, summon a nurse who could.

Not to belabor what I hope is obvious, but any humor I see in the shift change "experience" is all in retrospect. It was distinctly unfunny at the time. Yet, it can be survived.

I am fortunate in that my overall health has been very good and I have been hospitalized only once since that initial time. It wasn't until January 1994, almost three years after I had the tracheotomy and went on the ventilator. I was told that three years was an unusually lengthy period between hospitalizations for people with ALS. I certainly hadn't complained about missing the place! Now, however, a slight case of pneumonia — the killer of many an ALS patient because we cannot clear our lungs — and multiple bronchial infections had caught up with me. I spent nearly two weeks in ICU this time, while my doctor, in consultation with others, sought the right combination and dosages of antibiotics to treat my new ailments without aggravating any of the old ones. After innumerable IVs, pills, shots, blood tests, and X-rays, I was pronounced fit and allowed to go home.

Two things made this hospital stay quite a bit more difficult than the first. One was that I had learned volumes about my care by then. I knew when I needed to be suctioned, how I should be positioned, when it was time to "eat," and approximately eleven zillion other idiosyncratic items. The result of this expanded knowledge? I was more demanding. We finally had to rig up the alarm system that was a lifesaver at home because it allowed Judy to be my caregiver and still get things done, even take a nap, in other parts of the house. I could trigger a doorbell chime with my eyebrows and it worked well in the hospital — except when the sensor in the headband accidentally got moved so the alarm was overactive or, worse, inactive.

Second, I definitely chose the wrong day to be sick enough to go to the hospital. On the other hand, it was also precisely the right day. It was January 17, the day of the destructive Northridge earthquake that cost 60-some people their lives, ruined countless homes and businesses, and devastated my former university. We were lucky to have only minor structural damage but the house was an extraordinary mess. Everything was on the floor, dressers, TVs, lamps, photographs and paintings from the walls, dishes, glasses, cereal, all of my considerable library of books, papers from files, soccer balls, and other memorabilia. It was appalling. As I said, facetiously, to Scott Harris, columnist for the Los Angeles Times, I went to the hospital because "I couldn't deal with the cleanup."

There were other, more important advantages in going to the hospital on that particular day, aside from the fact that I needed to be hospitalized right away. The primary one was that the hospital had electricity while our home didn't. Two backup batteries would keep my ventilator running for 20 to 24 hours but there was no way to operate the suction machine, the humidifier or the PulmoAide for asthma treatments, all of which I needed regularly. (Since then, we have purchased our own generator; that gives us a much greater sense of security.) There were also important disadvantages, the chief among them being that almost everyone, including the ICU nurses, was preoccupied with the earthquake above all else. This was only natural as so many of them had had their lives turned virtually upside down and inside out by the disaster. Just as naturally, however, the nurses' general state of distraction also created some very irritating and unpleasant, but ultimately surmountable, problems. Most of the time, I found most of them to have less patience and shorter attention spans than they had demonstrated in the more normal circumstances of three years earlier. These conditions were, and are whenever I encounter them, more than a little frustrating for a person who can't speak and for whom communicating is a slow and somewhat tedious process (for both parties). Their powers of concentration and observation were similarly affected. I even had one experienced nurse finally respond to the shrill ventilator alarm — which meant that I was not getting air; this time because the tube bringing me air from the vent had popped off my trach and was lying uselessly on my chest — only to press the 30-second alarm silencer button and zoom out of the room without doing anything to solve the problem (i.e., giving me air). Truly astonishing! (Within a minute of the resumption of the alarm's wail, a different and more focused nurse came in, saw the problem immediately, and hooked me back up. It was nice to breathe again.)

Home Nurses

The real adventure was just beginning, however, when I arrived home that first time with my new tubes and assorted equipment. Talk about a shift change! We anticipated a somewhat rocky transition from the relative security of the hospital and, frankly, it was a bit scary, especially for Judy. (I was still pretty much in my own world, just pleased as punch to be present.) We were novices at all of this, green rookies, and now we were on our own. It was intimidating.

Being on our own meant being dependent on individual nurses and caregivers, not a staff of them within a hospital setting. Moreover, we either had to hire them ourselves or rely on a nursing agency. Our insurance covered, on average, a little over two 8-hour shifts per day so we could afford to hire "real" nurses, R.N.s and L.V.N.s who were trained on ventilators, through an agency. With Mario working five such shifts a week, I had care almost around the clock and Judy only had to do an occasional fill-in shift as my caregiver.

My experience with these professional nurses was decidedly mixed. On the one hand, I never ceased to marvel at the unending stream of people of questionable competence that the agency sent into my life. Some of them deserve special mention a little later. On the other, I had a substantial number of good, competent nurses, including some absolutely excellent ones. In this last category, I think fondly of Angel and David, Sandy and Agnes. And Earl, too. They had several admirable qualities in common, especially unusually high degrees of skills and caring, a critical combination for a nurse. They were also very patient in communicating with me. They even helped me with the Slugs, my fantasy baseball team!

All of these nurses came with interesting "stories," ranging from fascinating backgrounds to diverse and equally fascinating interests. Earl, for example, is a folk-rock musician as well as a licensed nurse. He plays the guitar and sings, writes music, and performs at local clubs. When his long hair is tied back, he is a nurse; when his locks are unfurled, he becomes a folk singer. And, he is very good at both. One evening, Earl and his girlfriend, a fine musician in her own right, came over and played terrific music for us for an hour and a half. When the concert ended, he rubber-banded his hair into a ponytail and, voila, was transformed back into my nurse for that night! Earl was also a voracious reader and we often discussed books we had read. Although he was only a part-time nurse for me, Earl and I became friends.

Beth, my regular, full-time night nurse for a lengthy period, occupies first place in my personal Hall of Fame for nursing excellence. One reason for that is we got to know each other quite well over the course of those months. We liked and respected one another and shared many of the same interests. A second reason is that I thought Beth embodied the qualities of the ideal nurse. Perhaps my feelings in this regard are expressed most clearly in this letter of recommendation I wrote for her shortly before she moved to Bakersfield.

To Whom It May Concern:

Beth S. has been my full-time night nurse for more than a year and a half. (She was part-time for two months prior to that.) She is an outstanding nurse in every respect.

Her nursing skills are excellent. She is knowledgeable, takes initiative, and is sensitive to my needs. She has been my primary nurse and I have always had complete confidence in her. She communicates very well, including with alphabet charts and the like. (I have ALS and am paralyzed, on a ventilator, and cannot speak.) She is extraordinarily dependable: she hardly missed a shift in all that time even with her long commute. Finally, she has a wonderful sense of humor and is a delightful person to be around.

As you can probably tell, I can't say enough about Beth both as a nurse and as a person.

Sincerely, Robert Horn

Oh yes, there is one more thing. It was also Beth who introduced me to and educated me in my newest love: country music. I have always loved classical music, especially Mozart, but sometimes I am more in the mood for Lorrie, Trisha, Willie, Mary, Vince, or Suzy. I know that Wolfgang would be appalled but it's great stuff!

There are, of course, two sides to every coin. For every good nurse there were at least two who were not so good. I must admit, right at the outset of this discussion, that the quality of a nurse, like beauty, is very much in the eye of the beholder. (Speaking of beauty, I had one nurse who was putting in extra hours to pay for what she called a "boob job," that is, a breast enlargement. On her first day back, she immediately and proudly showed me her new profile. I had to admit that it was quite impressive.) Each patient is different, with his or her own idiosyncrasies. Consequently, the "fit" with particular nurses will vary widely. One person's perfect example of incompetence may be another's Florence Nightingale.

That disclaimer having been made, I would like to think that most of the ones I have labeled as incompetents would be similarly regarded by most people in my situation. I mean, what else do you call night nurses, hired specifically to be alert for when you needed something because you could only signal to them with your eyes, who sleep more (just a slight exaggeration) than you do?! I had an abundance of these, more than I can count, including many who swore that they never slept on the job.

What else can you call "Jane" who was so obsessed with taking notes on me that she managed to ignore the actual me for about seven hours of her eight-hour shift? She did little but wrote much, beginning the instant she walked in the door. What she was basing her voluminous notes on, I cannot imagine. Maybe she was secretly working on a novel. And what about "Ronald"? He was a real piece of work. His obsession with two things, his biceps and chewing on a toothpick, made him blissfully and arrogantly oblivious to the world around him. He once wandered through the house for 10 minutes with a used bedpan, flexing all the way, apparently wondering, with apologies to MacBeth, "Is this a bedpan I see before me? If so, what the hell do I do with it?" Get a life, dude!

Perhaps my "favorite" among all the "winners" I have had was the first, "Dizzy Lizzy." My experience with her would have been funnier had we not been so dependent on her; she accompanied me home from the hospital and seemed to be the main link to my survival. The problem was that she didn't know anything. Well, that's not entirely fair. She may have known a great deal — it was just that most of it was out of date. She had been summoned out of retirement by the nursing agency we originally signed on with specifically to handle my case. She must have retired shortly after the Korean War; she appeared to be that old. Also, she knew precious little about my ventilator and, for the first several weeks at home, we had constant crises with which she didn't know how to cope. Use of the manual means of having me breathe, the reliable but demanding ambu-bag, was a regular, almost daily occurrence. She was very good at one thing, the art of scavenging — we came home with a ton of freebie tubing, urinals, bedpans, and other assorted equipment that she'd managed to talk the hospital out of. All in all, she was a nice person but, unfortunately, for someone with my needs, that just isn't enough.

A Crime

I want to report a crime. At least, I think it was, and is, criminal. It is a crime of the long-running sort. It began on August 1, 1993, and continues to this day. I do not know, exactly, who the perpetrators are and I am not sure what their punishment should be. Boiling in oil is a trifle extreme but definitely in the ballpark. What about a good, old-fashioned flogging? Perhaps they could be shipped to Singapore to receive a couple of dozen strokes of the rattan. Better yet, they should be sentenced to spend, say, two or three months on a ventilator with zero professional nursing care.

Now that I have revealed my biases and expressed my sense of outrage, an explanation is in order. In early 1993, we were notified that I would be eligible for Medicare beginning in August. We assumed, secure in our radiant naïveté, that this was good news since I then would be covered by two health insurance policies, my original one with Blue Shield and now also Medicare. Judy began making calls to find out what additional benefits I would be receiving. To our astonishment and growing consternation, we gradually discovered that there would be no extra benefits. Instead, there would be cuts in the benefits I had been getting!

We didn't believe it! There had to be some mistake or misunderstanding. Surely, Judy's inquiries would eventually unearth someone who would fight through the bureaucratese and straighten it all out. Despite countless telephone calls to Blue Shield, Medicare, my doctor, and even an advocate for Medicare patients, she failed to turn up such a rescuer.

The gist of my personal "new world order," to borrow a phrase from former President George Bush, was that, as of August first, I would be nurseless. My insurance would no longer cover home nursing shift care.

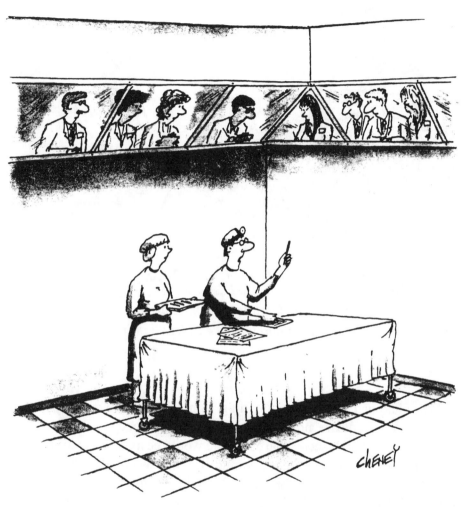

"Next, I will use a medium-point roller-ball pen with black ink and, on the anterior side of the upper-left quadrant, two centimetres below the binding staple, begin detailing in bold print the patient's previous medications and treatments relating to present indications for procedure and treatment, as required on this particular health-insurance form."

Drawing by Cheney; ©1995 *The New Yorker Magazine*, Inc.

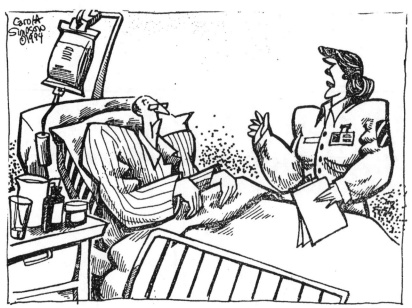

"The company has cut its healthcare contributions by 25%. What part of your body would you like to leave uninsured?"

Cartoon by Carol Simpson.

Where I had had two nurses providing 16 hours of care every day of the week before Medicare, now I would have no nurses and not a single hour of care on any day! It seems that Medicare would be my primary insurance coverage and BS (Blue Shield) would become secondary. That meant that BS would help pay for the deductible on any service Medicare provided. HOWEVER, it also meant that BS would not cover anything that Medicare didn't. And, since Medicare coverage, for some inexplicable reason, does not include shift care, BS doesn't either.

Nurseless in Northridge! It was not that my medical condition had changed in any way. I had neither recovered nor died. I hadn't even made progress toward either of those extremes. My health had been pretty much on a plateau since emerging from the hospital two years earlier and I continued to need qualified, licensed nursing care to keep it that way. Suddenly and arbitrarily, such care was taken from me. I still fail to see any rationale for that whatsoever. And I am still outraged. Maybe boiling in oil is, after all, not too extreme for those responsible.

Does the health care system in this country need to be reformed? From my individual perspective, it certainly does!

Caregivers

Another shift change! This one exceeded in magnitude the tremor that struck on my arrival home from the hospital. No more Beth. No more Earl or Angel or Dave. No more any of the other good nurses I had had. Naturally, it was good riddance to the incompetents, the weeds among the flowers, so to speak. But, to carry the metaphor a bit further, Judy and I knew we were now entering an untended garden where the weeds would greatly outnumber the flowers. "Caregivers," not qualified, licensed nurses. Pigs in a poke?

Of course, we could always hire most of the good nurses out of our own pocket. We would have to go through the agency, however, and at more than $30 an hour, that was far too pricey. We would have to venture into that garden ourselves and attempt to find the flowers among the weeds.

Enough of that metaphor already! What I mean to say is that we would have to advertise, interview, and hope to get lucky. We also would have to do a lot of training (ventilator, suctioning, feeding, etc., etc.) which would be the key. A host of unknowns.

Our efforts produced mixed results, as you might imagine. On the plus side, we did find a reliable, trainable (up to a point) person who stayed with us for a year and a half. On the negative side of the ledger, we invested considerable time, energy and money training some people who stayed for only a brief time. One woman worked one day after being trained before leaving town for unspecified reasons!

This wasted training is among our greatest frustrations. But there are others, too. One is the sheer expense of having to pay for round-the-clock care on our own with no help from either of my wonderful insurance policies. It's a substantial drain. Another frustration is the quality of my care. Most of the time, it is inferior to the care I received when I had "real" nurses. My new caregivers don't suction as well, can't make me as comfortable and have less knowledge of the ventilator. Moreover, there are serious questions about their ability to respond in a emergency. It is an insecure and unpleasant feeling.

Aggravating this problem is the fact that we hired some people who turned out to be of, shall we say, varying degrees of incompetence. Not surprisingly, we have been subjected to a higher proportion of these than we were in our earlier situation. One was awesomely lazy, never doing more than the minimum, very often less. He also became enraged and rude when suggestions were made on ways to improve his job performance. The last straw for another was when she, unbelievably, managed to cut my gastric tube in two with a pair of scissors. A first time for everything, I guess! (And the last, I hope!)

Some of my night nurses seemed to "work" mainly to catch up on their sleep. One of these evidently decided one night that a chair wasn't comfortable enough for a really good sleep. So he stretched out on the floor to indulge in some serious snoozing. When I woke up some time later, I was very uncomfortable and needed to be turned onto my other side. "Juan," who, incidentally, had been a physician in his native country, didn't seem to be anywhere around. After 10 minutes or so of getting increasingly angry with my absentee caregiver, I was actually relieved when the air tube happened, as it does occasionally, to pop off my trach. I wasn't able to breathe but I knew that the loud alarm on the ventilator would soon begin and that surely would get his attention wherever he was and whatever he was doing. I was wrong, almost fatally so. The alarm started ringing and there was still no sign of him. One minute. Two minutes. How could he be so slow? I remember hoping that he was not profoundly deaf. At four minutes, I began to get really concerned. I didn't know how long I could continue somehow taking these micro-mini-breaths. Where the hell was the jerk? At six minutes, fighting off the urge to panic, I figured he was never going to show up. I prayed for a miracle. After more than seven minutes with no artificial ventilation, one occurred: I watched in disbelief as Juan rose, Lazarus-like, from the floor of my study, ran over and reattached me. I will never know what woke him from his deep sleep at that particular moment, but I figure it had to be God.

It is difficult to fire someone whom you have spent considerable time training. That particular Sleeping Beauty was fired. On the spot. And with absolutely no difficulty or regret.

On a lighter note, we employed for three months a very assertive Egyptian Christian evangelist. To the extreme, it seemed to me. For example, when Judy was trying to get him to commit to the schedule before she went on a well-deserved vacation to visit her Mom in Buffalo, all he could say was "If it's God's will." Come on! And my personal favorite: in the middle of a simple procedure that he can't do and is overwhelmed by, he would inform me that "Jesus loves you." I always felt like telling him that I know that but, at this particular moment, I wish he could change my shirt.

A final major frustration of being nurseless and dependent on relatively unqualified caregivers is the immense additional burden it has placed on Judy. She is saddled with a great amount of extra paperwork and bears the brunt of the newly necessary interviewing and training processes. Even more significant, she has had to become a full-time caregiver — in addition to her regular, full-time job directing the preschool at the Methodist church in Westwood. Her new responsibility is necessitated by a combination of the lack of quality caregivers, especially for the hours we need them, and our desire to reduce our already astronomical expenditures for my care. Currently, on an average week, Judy is my caregiver for one morning, three afternoons, four evenings, and two nights. A total of 52 hours! That's a lot. Whenever I read about other ALS patients who have fully or even partially covered care, I am envious. That situation is the way it should be. In comparison, our situation, so to speak, really stinks.

Less care for monumentally more money with a much greater burden on my wife. Unfair? Unjust? Unconscionable? All of those and more. Thank you Blue Shield and Medicare.

There has been a saving grace throughout these months of unpleasantness. Actually, there have been two. Judy and Mario. Together they provide more than half of my care and both are very knowledgeable, caring, skilled, able to communicate, patient, and sensitive to my needs. Thank God for them.

8

REACHING WITHOUT ARMS

I have no arms.

Well, that's only figuratively, not literally, true. I do have arms but they are useless, except for filling out shirtsleeves. I have hands, too, but they are equally worthless and good only for cosmetic purposes. I remember longingly what those hands and arms used to be able to do, simple things, normal things: hug my wife, hold our children when they were babies and play with them as they got older, shoot a basketball, write, dress myself, shave or brush my teeth or hair, type on a computer, swing a tennis racket, hold a bridge hand, raise a margarita (without salt, of course) to my lips, touch, feel. Now I can only, with dexterous help, touch and feel but can do none of the others at all — with the notable exception of being able to use the computer with my foot. The frustrations this causes are multiple, constant, and endless. I can't even organize my notes and papers, much less shuffle them!

By no means am I implying that I consider myself to be worse off than other people with the same or other disabilities and diseases. If you have to have a disability or terminal illness, who can say which one of the many different kinds would be "preferable"? I certainly wouldn't be so presumptuous. For instance, would it be "better" to be paralyzed or blind? Since I have never been blind, I don't know. One of the books I read about the disability of blindness (see Bibliography) contained a candid argument for the greater disadvantages of sightlessness. The author complained that being blind robbed him of one of the great pleasures of sex, the visual. I have no doubt of this. But, as he admits, the essence of sex is tactile. I do not want to be blind but "you can look but you can't touch" detracts significantly from the joys of sexual intimacy.

The federal government, however, is willing to make just such a distinction. Congress, with the support of the executive branch, has written into law a differentiation between blindness and other disabilities. And the Supreme Court recently upheld the law by letting stand a lower court ruling against a quadriplegic man. By law, blind people who receive Social Security disability benefits can earn as much as $940 a month without losing those benefits while people with other disabilities can only earn up to $500. The quadriplegic in this case had earned $50 over his limit (by typing with his toes!), still well below the maximum for the sightless, and was denied further benefits and ordered to repay a substantial sum for past ones. Talk about a disincentive to work, to reach! The law strikes me as bizarre and I fail to see the logic behind its discrimination. Fact continues to be stranger than fiction!

One thing I do know: for me, a physical disability is preferable to a mental one. In This Far and No More, an ALS victim, who eventually succeeded in obtaining assistance to end her life, discusses the relative "merits" of ALS and Alzheimer's. Although her internal debate remains inconclusive, she writes wistfully of a disease where you would not be aware of your steady physical decline. Not me. My progressive deterioration was frustrating and depressing in the extreme but I'll still take that over losing my capacity to reason, to analyze, or to remember. For, as the remarkable Dan Quayle — remember him? — misspoke in one of his innumerable verbal gaffes, "What a waste it is to lose one's mind." Indeed!

My mind, such as it is, has been my salvation. It still is. I am no brilliant thinker but I do enjoy the world of the mind, which is only appropriate for someone who has spent his entire life in school, either studying or teaching — and always learning. I am comfortable there because there is so much more to learn, so many things I am interested in and curious about, an unceasing flow of books I am anxious to delve into and a number of topics I would like to write about. My mind is my means of setting goals and striving to achieve them.

In the late spring of 1994, my college fraternity magazine published an article about me. As a result, I received several letters and faxes from fraternity brothers with whom I had not been in contact for a full three decades. I enjoyed their news and appreciated their words of encouragement. One has become a regular correspondent, sending me letters, cards, and pictures of his family. One card in particular struck me as so symbolic of my situation that I asked Mario to tape it to one of my sliding closet doors next to my bed. It serves as a reminder and source of inspiration. On the front was a beautiful photograph of a man, in silhouette, climbing a sheer rock-face with clouds below him and other mountains bathed in sunlight in the background. The inside had been blank and Dave wrote just a single word, "Reach!" With the exclamation point! I like to think of myself as reaching: to learn, to enjoy, to love and, perhaps most importantly, to contribute. Although I have to do it without the use of my arms, I can still reach. Thanks, Dave.

"The Columnist"

Two and a half years before embarking on the relatively mammoth project of writing this book, I did something equally brave and significant for me at the time. I reached. And it was a substantial reach, too, at least for me.

By the beginning of 1992, I was growing restless. It was less than a year after the trach, vent, and all that but my health was stable and I had regained a lot of my energy. I felt the need to do something more. I was reading up a storm with my page turner but wasn't communicating what I learned with anyone. I was also writing, but only letters. Maybe I could combine these two loves of mine and produce something that would be of interest to others. But what audience to address? An article for a professional journal, of which I had done a couple of dozen in my prior, "normal" life, seemed far too ambitious — both because of the length and the fact that I didn't have the necessary research materials at my, so to speak, fingertips. I needed to undertake a project of more modest and fun scale.

Finally, I hit upon what I thought was a fairly off-the-wall idea. I proposed to Dave and Maria, my good friends and pastors of our Methodist church in Northridge, that I be allowed to write a monthly column for the weekly church newsletter. The articles would be about various aspects of world affairs, particularly developments in the former Soviet Union, and would include brief reviews of new, relevant books. I outlined my plans for the first six columns and explained that their tone would be informal rather than academic. They would attempt to provide some perspective to better understand contemporary international events, raise issues and questions, and perhaps provoke some discussion. I admitted to Dave and Maria that I had selfish motives, such as a sense of self-fulfillment, for the request as well as more altruistic ones.

That proposal turned out to be one of the best things I ever did. Its coming to fruition greatly aided my psychological recovery. I will be forever grateful to Dave and Maria for their immediate and warmly enthusiastic "thumbs up." Maria's only question was "When do we begin?" Since I had been chomping at the bit for some time, I started flicking my eyebrows the next day! Of course, I had a number of apprehensions about the project in spite of my own enthusiasm. Could I actually accomplish it, physically? Did I really have anything significant and/or interesting to say? What would the reaction be? Would members of the congregation like it, find it of interest?

The answers to my questions have been resoundingly in the affirmative. After more than 3 years and close to 50 columns, I must be, as the saying goes, doing something right! The first one, which explained the intention and purposes of the columns and reviewed Bette Bao Lord's wonderful book on China, *Legacies*, appeared in February 1992. My most recent column, a discussion of why President Clinton should go to Moscow to participate in ceremonies commemorating the 50th anniversary of the end of World War II in Europe, was published in April 1995. The first 15 to 20 (I lost count, my old computer program couldn't save them, and I am too lazy to dig through my files) were written with my eyebrows and the last 28 (the new computer keeps track) with my foot. I have written on international politics, American and Russian foreign policy, Russian and Malaysian politics, Soviet and Russian history, and reviewed at least a couple dozen books. I also wrote several articles about my personal experiences of coping. The columns are short by academic standards, usually between 400 and 500 words (about one single-spaced, typed page).

The response to these columns has been positive, enthusiastic and, therefore, extremely gratifying. I have received dozens of notes complimenting me on various articles and am routinely stopped at church by people who want to discuss a particular one or just to tell me that they had enjoyed it. The significance for me of this writing and the reaction to it is hard to overestimate. I feel like I am again contributing to something beyond myself. I am making a difference, however small, and that is a priceless feeling. I suppose it comes down to a reaffirmation of my sense of self-esteem which was under siege because of my helplessness and dependency.

Limitations and Perspective

My area of expertise and teaching responsibility as a college professor was international relations with a specialization in the Soviet Union and Soviet foreign policy. Several common themes ran through all the courses I taught. I emphasized — ad nauseam, I am sure, to my students — one of these in particular because it is crucial to understanding how and why states in the international arena behave and interact with each other. It is also an essential consideration in policy making. At least it should be — see, for example, the discussion in Robert S. McNamara's book on American policy in Vietnam, *In Retrospect: The Tragedy and Lessons of Vietnam*. It is equally important, I think, in interpersonal relations. That theme or issue is perception.

What the study of perception in world politics teaches is that so-called "objective reality" is actually the subjective perception and interpretation of situations, events, interests, and other actors by various decision makers in every state and other entity. States pursue their interests based on their particular perception or view of reality. That, in turn, is shaped by the complex interplay between a whole range of factors and considerations, including geography, economic strengths and weaknesses, history, ideology, military capabilities, the political situation, and various intangibles such as national character. All of this means that in order to understand why the old Soviet Union or the United States, or Malaysia, Israel or Ecuador, took a certain foreign policy action, you have to put yourself in "the other guy's shoes." You have to see the situation through his eyes, understand that state's perception, its perspective.

So what, you might well ask? Is this somehow relevant to the matter at hand or just some extraneous lecture pulled from a musty file? Simply put, the study of perception reminds us that there are different ways of looking at the same issue, event, problem, or situation. And this is true at all levels of life, from the global to the personal. The linkage between perception and living life is that we act on what we perceive. In other words, our perception, or perspective determines how we live. This makes the discussion relevant for my life, indeed for all of our lives.

What is my perspective, then, on my life? Not oversimplifying the question very much at all, it comes down to that old conundrum: do I see the glass as half full or half empty? Before the diagnosis of ALS, I had always viewed the glass as half full. I was an unabashed optimist, albeit tempered with a certain degree of realism. But how about now? Admittedly, there is not much to like, and a great deal to find intolerable, about my current situation. It is difficult, to say the least, living under the sentence of a terminal disease, knowing that I will not get better, only worse. I have to try to avoid reflecting on longer-term concepts of time, such as "never" or "forever." They are psychologically painful. Physically, I'm a mess. I can't do anything for myself, have virtually no workable muscles and can't move. It is frustrating and maddening to be so absolutely helpless and so totally dependent on others. If my head lolls to one side or the other, as it often does, it stays there unless and until someone notices and props it up again. If an arm slips off the armrest of the wheelchair, it will just dangle by my side until someone retrieves it. And I drool. More than is generally acceptable in polite society. I hate that! (One of the several unpleasant "fringe benefits" of my kind of ALS is that I am producing increased amounts of saliva at the same time that swallowing has become next to impossible.)

Among other things, I greatly miss eating. I loved to eat! I enjoyed just about every kind of food (except, of course, for peas which I am convinced were never intended for human consumption), especially various "ethnic" cuisines. Have you noticed how many food commercials there are on television? I have. They seem almost constant and they drive me nuts because I can still remember the taste of different foods. On the other hand, if I were suddenly cured and could eat, I'd probably go on a fast-food binge, balloon to 350 pounds, get clogged arteries, and have a heart attack!

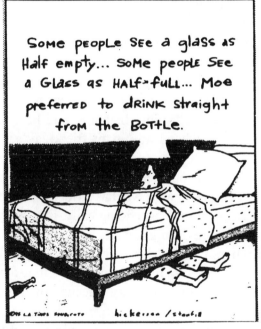

The Quigmans by Buddy Hickerson. ©1995, *Los Angeles Times Syndicate*. Reprinted by permission.

There is ample evidence to think the glass is now at least half empty. Well, it almost is, but not quite. There is more to life than physical ability. There are the mental, emotional, and spiritual abilities or worlds to consider as well. In these worlds, I haven't changed: I am still a vibrant, healthy, and independent person. I can think, reason and analyze, remember, read, write, learn and communicate. I can love, feel happiness and sadness, be enthusiastic, get angry, have highs and lows, feel joy. I can believe, hope and have faith. That adds up to an extensive list of things I can still "do" in spite of my disease.

There are even some things in my life that have actually improved. Not many, but a few. Anne Morrow Lindbergh, in her insightful Gift From The Sea, stresses the value of simplifying our overly busy and complicated lives. I have done that. True, it was forced on me but I am able to appreciate what she meant. My life is necessarily less hectic and my "schedule" has certainly been simplified. I have more time for reflection and contemplation. As a result, I think I understand some aspects of life a little better than I used to. I think I can reason and analyze a little better, too. An important part of this is that I have become a better listener. I had always regarded myself as an attentive and thoughtful listener but I am impressed at how much more I really hear now that I can't talk. Like everyone else, I had trouble listening and hearing — there's a significant difference — when I was, in my friend Jay's words, "flapping my gums."

This is not to say that I consider my current state of existence superior to my former one. I don't. No way! Nor has the disease been a dramatically life-altering experience for me psychologically. I feel very much like the same person I was before. It might make a good plot for a TV movie to say that I have been transformed by my confrontation with ALS, that my values and priorities have radically shifted, or that I have become a decidedly better person in some way because of the disease. But it wouldn't be true. I would gladly regain my ignorance, become a poor listener, and give up kicking the computer and page turner in exchange for the return of my physical abilities. Actually, naturally, I would like to have both but I would dearly love to be back in the classroom, work in the yard, pet the dogs, shoot baskets in the driveway, eat, travel to see our kids, and do a thousand other things I can no longer do.

This brings me back to the question of my overall perspective of my situation. I am convinced that what I have left is more valuable than what I have lost. I believe that the things I can do are more important than those I can't. The key for my psychological well-being is to focus on what I can do, my abilities, rather than on my disabilities and limitations. To dwell on the latter is to wallow in grief and self-pity. Such wallowing is, for me, sometimes unavoidable and occasionally even necessary. But to concentrate on the former is to invite optimism, achievement, and new opportunities.

All in all, I would say that the glass has lost some of its water but it is still half full.

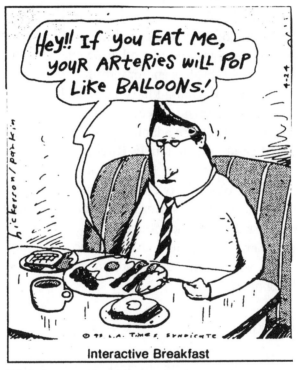

Interactive Breakfast

The Quigmans by Buddy Hickerson. ©1995, *Los Angeles Times Syndicate*. Reprinted by permission.

Aside: Feeling Russian

Perhaps I am imagining it or maybe I have just been studying Russia for too long a time, but in coping with this disease I sometimes see myself as Russian. I don't mean that I have "gone native," as that derogatory expression goes, but I do greatly admire a number of attributes of the Russian people, attributes that I think are relevant to my situation. Foremost among these is the Russians' ability to "endure": to endure centuries of political repression and tyranny, abject poverty, harsh and long winters, devastating wars, and foreign invasions. While I can't quite compare my enduring of ALS to these, they seem to have something in common. Like the Russians and like other people who choose to go on living despite severe disabilities and/or terminal illness, I am willing, as the cliché says, to "play the hand I have been dealt."

There are two other pertinent aspects of the Russian national character with which I identify. They are adaptation and compromise. Of course, these characteristics are not uniquely Russian but they are especially pronounced among peoples who have had to live under a totalitarian political system. For most of the twentieth century, and particularly during the nearly 30 years of Stalin's murderous rule, communism required Russians, even dissidents, to adapt and make compromises in order to survive. It is the same for people with disabilities. We, too, are forced to make adjustments, adaptations, and compromises to get on with life. After all, what's the choice?

The Power of Choice

In fact, people confronted with physical disability and terminal illness have, at least they SHOULD have, three basic choices: to die, to exist, or to live. I am not ready to die. And, as long as I continue to breathe, even with the aid of a machine, I will try to live life to the fullest extent possible rather than be content merely to exist. That's my choice.

Some time ago, I saw a report on CNN that left me disturbed and reflective. It was about the controversy surrounding the issue of doctor-assisted suicide in Canada, a complex and thought-provoking issue in its own right. What personalized it for me, though, was that the three people the report profiled who all wanted to end their lives were suffering from the same disease as I am, ALS. Moreover, the impact of the report was intensified by the condition of the patients. With varying difficulty, all could eat and talk and none was on a ventilator.

Since then, there have been several highly publicized cases of ALS patients seeking medical assistance to end their lives humanely and with some dignity. Most of these cases have been in Michigan, and have involved Dr. Jack Kevorkian. The November 1994 elections in Oregon increased the available options in that state for those ill enough to consider ending their lives. This new law is now in the courts under appeal. The moral, ethical, humanitarian, and legal issues and arguments swirling around these and other, similar cases are complicated and controversial. Some predict that the question of whether or not to legalize euthanasia will become the dominant social issue before the end of the century.

My choice, to go on living in spite of the disease, doesn't make me "better" or more "courageous" than those who opt for alternative solutions to the challenges they face. The personal struggles of people against life-threatening illnesses do not lend themselves to facile or self-righteous judgments. These are highly individual battles that depend on many factors, from personal outlook and philosophy, to the specific situation and circumstances of the patient, and, significantly, on the nature of the illness itself.

In considering ALS specifically, there are at least three major reasons to avoid being judgmental in the evaluation of how a particular victim of the disease reacts to it. For one, its symptoms vary dramatically from patient to patient; one person's experience with the disease is no guide to someone else's. For instance, one of the women in the CNN report suffered substantial physical pain. I have had considerable discomfort but minimal pain — other than, earlier, from falls or muscle cramps in my legs and, more recently, when a caregiver turns me awkwardly or some such thing.

Second, I greatly sympathize with those people who are in the earlier stages of the disease. As I have told Judy, for me "getting this way was worse than being this way." Much, much worse. The mental stress of

watching the progressive deterioration of your basic physical abilities —
loss of dexterity, falling, having trouble swallowing, losing your voice
— is enormous and exceptionally depressing. My situation now is
relatively secure. Much, much more secure.

Finally, the decision of whether or not to go on life support is an
intensely personal one. I made the right decision for me, but that is not to
suggest that my choice would be the appropriate one for everyone
confronted with a similar dilemma.

Compare my situation, for example, to that of Thomas Hyde. He was
the man with ALS who Dr. Kevorkian helped to end his life in August
1993. While I was in my mid-forties when I was diagnosed with the
disease, Mr. Hyde was in his twenties. And our occupations were also
quite dissimilar: mine was indoor-focused, college teaching, and his
was in the outdoors, in landscaping and construction. These m a j o r
differences mean that the impact of similar physical changes on each of
us would vary due to our different lifestyles. I would like to think that if
I had been in his position, I still would have chosen life — but I wasn't
so I can't truly know what my ultimate decision would have been.

All that said, I would still like to talk to those people who are seeking
to end their lives — and would have liked to talk to those who did. What
would I say? I would simply tell them that "there is life on a ventilator."
They would probably respond by asking me what good could that kind
of life be. Admittedly, it is often difficult. Compared to being "normal,"
the list of frustrations and "wants" is endless. For me, however, it is
good just to be alive! The positives outweigh the negatives (although, on
my periodic "bad" days, it seems not by a whole lot). I have to assess the
quality of my life in slightly different terms but it is still full of
opportunities, challenges, rewards, and joys. There are many things I am
curious about and interested in. I enjoy the richness, diversity, and
complexity of life. I want to see what my children do with their lives. I
have retained my 30-year fascination with Russia and with Asia,
particularly Southeast Asia. There are things I want to write about and
books I want to read. And, among other interests, I also want to continue
to "manage" my fantasy baseball team (even in the face of greedy strikes
and pathetic also-ran finishes every year). I suppose the bottom line is

what you do after going on the ventilator. I am fortunate in that many things that I love I can still do.

This doesn't mean I don't sometimes — like daily — bemoan my situation. I do (but, usually, only to myself). There are so many things I used to enjoy that I can no longer do. There are so many things I looked forward to doing that are now impossible.

In the beginning, I agonized over the "why me" question. I soon realized, however, how emotionally draining and generally unproductive that line of inquiry could prove to be. Moreover, I eventually discovered what seems to me to be the logical answer to the question: "Why not me?" I also admire the way Arthur Ashe, the late tennis great and humanitarian, dealt with the question in his struggle with AIDS. In his autobiography, *Days of Grace*, he explains that since he never asked the question when he was enjoying personal and professional success, he had no right to raise it now. This is a philosophy with which I fully concur.

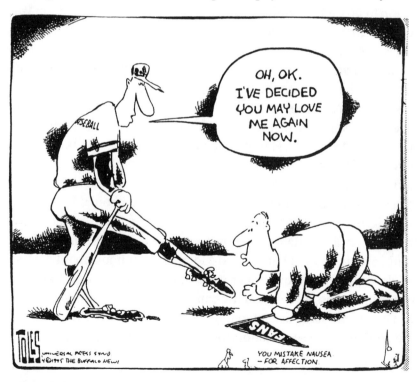

Toles ©1995 *The Buffalo News*. Reprinted with permission of UNIVERSAL PRESS SYNDICATE. All rights reserved.

I have also lamented the fact, and others have too, that "it just isn't fair." Of course it isn't. Unfortunately, as we all know, life is not "fair." I think about "fairness" when I read about children starving in Rwanda or being killed in random drive-by shootings in Los Angeles and other American cities. Compared to them and countless other examples, what reason could I possibly have to complain about "fairness"? I have a wonderful wife, three terrific children, a career I had found both challenging and enormously rewarding, plus I had traveled widely and coached youth soccer for many years. All these things I loved and embraced enthusiastically. No regrets. And yet, I suppose it's human nature always to want more. I know I do. I feel, arrogantly I admit, short-changed, robbed of a third of my life. There are so many things I wanted to do.

Enough bemoaning what was or what might have been.

The underlying point of all this is that I had a choice. I made a conscious decision to go on the ventilator and on with my life. The decision wasn't made by a doctor or anyone else but me. I even had two doctors offer me the option of ending my life painlessly. So, when I chose life, I knew there was an alternative available. I am very happy with the decision I made and I can live with the negatives, frustrations, and downs because I chose. My parents taught me that I had to live with the consequences of my decisions and, for me, the benefits of living far outweigh the costs just as I had expected. Having a choice is the key and makes all the difference in the world. It's as simple, and as complicated, as that!

I imagine that everyone who faces the debilitating and terminal nature of diseases like ALS would prefer to have such a choice. I support that. Dennis Kaye, in his book *Laugh, I Thought I'd Die*, says he does not want to go on a ventilator when it becomes necessary. I don't think he should have to. In This Far and No More, another book about a personal struggle with ALS, Emily Bauer wrote in her diary: "I don't know how anyone with access to a normal life can expect me to accept such a limited one. That others have accepted a drastically limited life does not mean that is the right course of action for me." I couldn't agree more!

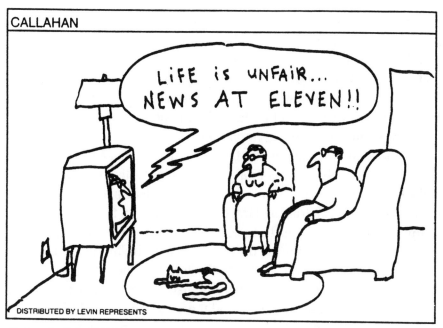

Cartoon by John Callahan.

This is not the time nor the place to launch into a full-blown discussion of the euthanasia issue. Suffice to say, I am in favor of legalizing euthanasia because that is the only way to provide terminally ill patients with an effective, legal choice regarding their future. I think such choice is vital. At the same time, however, I recognize that there are manifold legal and moral questions involved. There are two new books I am aware of that thoughtfully explore many of these questions: *Rethinking Life and Death* by Peter Singer and a new edition of *Suicide in America* by Herbert Hendin. When we have the technology to prolong life almost indefinitely, who decides when we die? What is needed is a thorough, public discussion of the issue.

Another Aside: Doctor-Bashing?

It would seem appropriate, and quite fashionable, to engage in some heavy-duty criticism of the medical profession at some point in this book.

Maybe it should have been a running theme throughout the book. Almost half the books discussed in the bibliography contain serious bashing. Physicians are criticized particularly for neglecting the mind part of the body-mind relationship, for concentrating on the disease while ignoring the person with the disease, for focusing on technology rather than people. In specific ALS cases, and perhaps for the profession in general, such criticism seems justified and important.

The problem with me as the basher is that I have hardly anyone to bash! Now, I freely confess to a potential bias in favor of doctors. My dad and my father-in-law were excellent physicians in every respect and my brother, a psychiatrist, and my brother-in-law, in family practice, are following in that tradition. The question of bias aside, I have nothing but praise and admiration for the doctors I have dealt with in the course of my seven-year battle with ALS. Well, there have been two exceptions. Both happened to be insensitive neurologists. Other than that pair, every doctor who has crossed my path, and there have been a lot of them, has impressed me as understanding of my situation, caring and sensitive, as well as highly skilled. Gordon Dowds, my "pulmonary man" and primary care physician, and neurologists Michael Graves (unfortunate name) of UCLA and Richard Smith of La Jolla are especially shining examples. Maybe I have just been lucky.

I don't know if an "aside to an aside" is proper or not but here is one anyway. I was never more impressed with hospital personnel — doctors, nurses and other staff — than I was on the morning of the 1994 Northridge earthquake. As you may remember, it was on that morning, in the aftermath of the quake, that I decided that I needed to go to the hospital to be checked for what turned out to be multiple upper respiratory infections. Everybody who could get to the hospital that chaotic morning was there! It was outstanding! In the parking lot, we bumped into (figuratively speaking, that is) one of my favorite respiratory therapists and she rolled me straight into a cubicle in the overflowing emergency room. Within 20 minutes all three of my main physicians had been in to see me and one of them admitted me to the hospital a short time later. My Ear, Nose and Throat doctor was in the next cubicle stitching up people who had suffered cuts because of the earthquake. Nurses we knew were everywhere. All this was despite the fact that many of these people had sustained considerable, in some cases major to the extent of total loss, damage to their own homes. Impressive indeed!

Hope

ALS doesn't leave much room for hope. The progress that has been made since the disease was first identified in the middle of the last century has not been impressive or encouraging. In fact, most of the research and notable progress has concerned familial ALS, a hereditary form of the disease which accounts for only a small proportion of ALS cases. We still don't know what causes the disease or how to treat, arrest or improve it. A cure? Forget it!

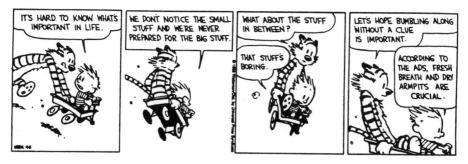

Calvin and Hobbes. Watterson. Dist. by Universal Press Syndicate. Reprinted with permission. All rights reserved.

There is, however, another, brighter, more hopeful side to this coin. The most significant is that the greatest advances in ALS research have been achieved in the last 10 or 15 years. There are several clinical trials of different drugs currently underway or recently concluded. Ten years ago, there were none! Moreover, researchers are getting much closer to isolating the cause, actually the causes plural, of ALS. (See *The New*

York Times, May 9, 1995.) It's a new and exciting era for ALS researchers and neurologists. And a more encouraging and hopeful one for ALS patients. New adaptive devices that will enrich the life of someone in my situation may be invented tomorrow; five years ago, for example, technology did not exist which would allow me to write down these thoughts as I am able to do today. A drug that can arrest the progression of ALS or some other disease may be discovered next week. Next month a cure may be found. Who knows?

There is still room for hope. Many people believe that where hope exists, life can flourish. I agree but I think the converse is also true: Where there is life, there is always hope. In the meantime, I am an admirer of Don Quixote; I can identify with his willingness, as sung in Man of La Mancha, to "fight the unbeatable foe."

This is exactly what I have chosen to do.

IN PLACE OF
A CONCLUSION

Getting On with the Business of Living

My situation is comparable to that of an infant. We are equally helpless and equally dependent on others for our survival. Completely dependent. There are differences, of course. For one, I can, with difficulty, communicate my needs. On the other hand, the infant will become less dependent and eventually independent. I won't.

If I am going to think in terms of analogies, however, I prefer to go in a different direction. I would probably draw from the world of sports. Baseball would be good in my case. For instance, I have compared my life to a baseball team that has rallied to send the big game into extra innings. My life was comfortable, happy, fulfilling and, by my definition, successful. I was well ahead in the "game of life" through the seventh inning. The score was, say, 10-3, not a perfect game by any means but a sizable lead. Then I ran into serious problems with the onset of ALS. The eighth and ninth innings were disastrous and I entered the bottom of the ninth behind by a run. I managed to tie the game up, not with anything so dramatic as a home run but rather with an infield single, a stolen base, a sacrifice bunt, and a sacrifice fly. A scratch run, eked out by determination and the sacrifices by other people. Since then, March of 1991, these same two factors have enabled me to keep the game going for all these extra innings.

I like that simple analogy drawn from the everyday world for many reasons. Alas, it does have a significant flaw. It says that the outcome of the game is still in doubt, that the winner has yet to be determined. I object! I think I have already won this game. After all, I have enjoyed a rich and meaningful life with manifold blessings and continue to do so, even with my limitations. What else is there?

Sticking with baseball, a better analogy would be a doubleheader. An *unscheduled* doubleheader. I am thinking of the famous statement by Ernie Banks, the great Hall of Fame shortstop for the Chicago Cubs: "It's a beautiful day for baseball. Let's play two." I am playing two. I "won" the regularly scheduled game and, thanks to the ventilator, I am able to play this extra game. My enthusiasm for the unscheduled part of the doubleheader is not quite as great as Ernie's, whose zeal for the game was unmatched, but it's close. It is a beautiful day for the game of life and I am very happy to still be a participant.

In the game of life, it all comes down to how you keep score. If dying is losing, then we are all losers because we are all terminal. The game makes no sense. A far more meaningful basis for scorekeeping is the *quality* of life. Quality rather quantity or longevity. How do you assess quality? That very much depends on perception and personal perspective.

Quality is *not* determined by the normal bumps in the road which everyone experiences. In life, as the bumper sticker crudely but truthfully states, "Shit happens." Indeed it does! Mary Chapin Carpenter sings about the fact of life that sometimes you're the bat and sometimes you're the ball, that "sometimes you're the windshield and sometimes you're the bug." I have always liked the way that Judy's brother, Don, has expressed this basic truth: "Sometimes you eat the bear and sometimes the bear eats you." If you can't deal with the naturally occurring and inevitable downs, the game of life is not for you. You have to accept the bad with the good. Most of us have learned to do that. We have also learned that, as I told the girls on my soccer teams, the test of our character is how we respond to adversity and setbacks, losses, disappointments, and defeats.

My response to ALS has run the emotional gamut. And gauntlet. I have experienced despair, fear, resignation, anger, and the dashing of unrealistic hopes, amid a torrent of emotions. Some time ago, I arrived at an acceptance of my condition and of reality. My "psychological problems" now relate not so much to my physical limitations or the fatal nature of my disease per se, but rather to the burden I am on others. Especially on Judy. She denies it but I feel I am and it bothers me a lot.

On the other hand, I have been surrounded by so much unconditional love that it is overwhelming. Especially by Judy. But from so many others, too. My favorite passage in the Bible has long been from First Corninthians. Paul wrote to the church in Corinth, "If I speak in tongues of men and of angels, but have not love, I am a noisy gong or a clanging cymbal." Well, no gongs or cymbals here! Family and friends are the instruments and reflection of God's love and I am continuously uplifted by them. They demonstrate that, as Paul further wrote, "Love bears all things, believes all things, hopes all things, endures all things." That passage means even more to me now. It has become very personal and very real.

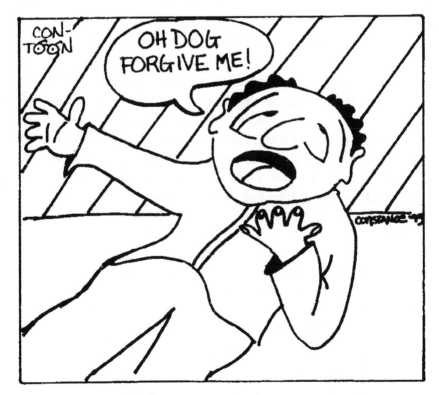

BOB's DYSLEXiA KEPT HiM OUT OF HEAVEN

Contoons by Constance Houck

Where does all this leave me? Fundamentally, I believe that I am as close as I will ever be to achieving, or being granted, the serenity so eloquently expressed in the "Serenity Prayer" by Reinhold Niebuhr: "God give us the grace to accept with serenity the things that cannot be changed, the courage to change the things which should be changed, and the wisdom to distinguish one from the other."

I love that prayer! I also think it fits my situation absolutely perfectly. I HAVE to accept my disabilities if I am going to keep on living. There is no alternative, except, I suppose, insanity and I am not quite ready for that. I also NEED to be able to distinguish what I can change in my life from what I can't. Finally, I definitely REQUIRE the courage to do all that I am capable of in my life. All of this adds up to the need to focus on things I can do and not to dwell on those I can't.

All three parts of the "Serenity Prayer" are essential to my ability to cope with my disease. The most intriguing part for me, however, is the one about having the courage to seek change, to strive, and to reach. That represents my biggest challenge and, within the context of the disease, I welcome it. Simplistically put, "Not guts, no glory." Challenges are a necessary, indeed vital, ingredient for living, for life. I certainly wouldn't have chosen ALS for my challenge, but that's the one I have.

My doctor, Gordon Dowds, has an interesting take on this struggle. After I told him of my intention to write this book, he responded with a lengthy fax that contained a number of insights, examples, and this viewpoint:

> My perspective is that we all start out living in a very small circle. Wrapped in a blanket, covered in a crib, we begin. The expansion of our circle is easy — we explode as young adults. It is the contraction that is hard. We all some day must contract. It may be from the loss of beauty for the cheerleader. A crippling disease. A sudden catastrophe such as ALS or a stroke. The measure of the man is how rich do we make the small sphere that we will one day find ourselves enclosed within.

I agree and I am trying to enrich my diminished circle as much as possible in terms of my interests.

Harper Lee, in *To Kill a Mockingbird,* defines courage as knowing "you're licked before you begin but you begin anyway and you see it through no matter what." Well, ALS has licked me, just as it licks everyone it touches. But I am only physically beaten. My spirit, though battered a bit and somewhat bruised, survives and remains strong. I refuse to let ALS win that battle, too.

My chances for recovery are between infinitesimal and zero. I don't have time to get bogged down in thinking about that, however. I am just too busy with life. My period of grieving is long over and I have gotten on with the business of living. I am glad that I am still an active participant in this exciting business.

In the end, if I have to have a nasty disease, at least I have one named from someone with whom I am familiar. And a baseball giant at that! Actually, Gehrig was a Yankee, but he was also a giant.

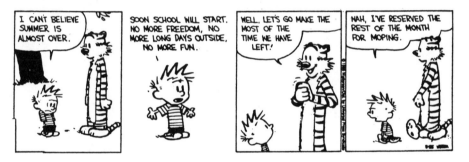

Calvin and Hobbes. Watterson. Dist. by Universal Press Syndicate. Reprinted with permission. All rights reserved.

Appendix

The Appendix contains several articles written about me that have appeared in the Los Angeles Times. They are included for the purpose of providing the reader with further information and clarification about my situation and outlook. They are factually accurate.

Also included is a joint, or "dialogue," sermon Rev. David Richardson and I gave at Northridge United Methodist Church. It puts my perspective in a broader context.

Finally, there is a sermon Judy and I delivered on Laity Sunday October 16, 1995 at the same church.

Los Angeles Times
January 20, 1993

AN INDOMITABLE FIGURE

BOB HORN LED CHATSWORTH GIRLS' SOCCER TEAM TO 2 CITY
TITLES, NOW HE BATTLES THE DEBILITATING EFFECTS OF LOU
GEHRIG'S DISEASE

By Kennedy Cosgrove
Special to *The Times*

Ask Bob Horn about the part he played in helping to found City Section girls' soccer in 1988, or why the team he coached, Chatsworth High, has won every City championship, and watch his eyebrows.

That's the only way Bob Horn can communicate. With his eyebrows.

Horn, 50, stricken since 1988 with amyotrophic lateral sclerosis — commonly known as Lou Gehrig's disease — has been unable to speak or voluntarily move any part of his body except his eyebrows for almost two years.

In the 1990-91 season — his second and last at the helm of the team — Horn coached from a wheelchair. Longtime friend Jack Sidwell served as an assistant as Chatsworth won its third consecutive City title. Coaching without Horn this season, Sidwell has led the top-seeded Chancellors (7-0) into the playoffs today against Bell.

Five years ago, Horn tirelessly lobbied City officials to start a girls' soccer program, in part so his daughter, Laura, whom he had coached in soccer since she was 6, would have an opportunity to play high school soccer.

In 1988, his efforts paid off. The year before Laura entered Chatsworth, City girls' soccer began.

Said Horn: "I was persistent and fairly obnoxious."

Actually, he doesn't <u>say</u> that. His wife, Judy, does. And it takes him more that three minutes to get that across to her.

***

When Horn wants to communicate, he raises his eyebrows to Judy. She seems to sense it.

"Do you want to add something?" Judy asks.

He raises his eyebrows. The left one moves only slightly. The right arches more, maybe a quarter-inch.

"One, two, three," Judy recites in a monotone, counting to seven, waiting for her husband to signal her.

She refers to a chart that consists of the alphabet neatly aligned in five rows of letters followed by two rows of five numerals. As Judy counts four, Bob arches his eyebrows.

The fourth row.

"P,Q,R,S..." Judy ticks off.

His eyebrow jumps.

"S." She writes it down.

The first letter is out of the way. Time for the second.

"One, two, three..."

The couple, married for 27 years, have shortcuts. Often she will need only one or two letters to guess the word. Usually she is right. If not, the painstaking process continues.

For a man who has traveled the world, served as a Cal State Northridge political science professor for nearly a quarter-century, earned a Fulbright scholarship and acted as a consultant for Rand Corp., it has reached this point.

For Bob Horn, who spent his life sharing himself and his ideas with others, communication now comes one letter at a time.

"It is very frustrating," he said. "I do better in writing than in person."

Horn has a special computer program and sensor keyed to his eyebrows that enables him to use his computer. Despite the effort simple communication now requires, he writes a monthly newsletter for his church.

"I think the key to communication is to respect your audience," he said. "And that hasn't changed."

But so much else has since he felt that first twinge in his upper left arm five years ago while riding his bicycle to work. It was the first symptom of the ordeal to come.

The twinges spread to his left leg. Doctors ruled out possible causes one by one. He traveled to Detroit in June, 1988, and the diagnosis was confirmed. ALS.

ALS poses few mysteries. The deterioration of the nerve cells that control muscular movement is well-documented and predictable. Motor control becomes increasingly difficult and then nonexistent. The abilities to speak and swallow are lost, and eventually the capacity to breathe. Every ALS sufferer knows the progression and the choice he must face — to be placed on a ventilator or die.

To choose the ventilator means a life of complete physical inaction, living with an active mind imprisoned in an unresponsive body. It is not an easy choice.

Bob Horn has always been a participant, living a life not only of action but of interaction.

A professor at CSUN for 22 years, he was no stodgy academician, whiling away his hours in solitary research.

He and George Brown, a fellow Northridge professor, put together a course in 1988 to illustrate Soviet-U.S. relations. Simulating political leaders coping with international crises, Horn's students took the position of the Soviet Politburo and Brown's that of the National Security Council.

"It was a fun class that everyone got involved with," said his former teaching assistant, Steve Hirsch. "He had a long list of people who wanted to get into his classes. He is one of those rare professors who really cared about his students."

Horn introduced a model United Nations program at CSUN in 1972 that still exists and served as the program's adviser for nearly 20 years. He often invited his students to his Canoga Park home for dinner.

"Unlike some teachers, I always liked my students," Bob said.

Said Judy: "He believed in letting the kids get to know him better and the family better and letting them get to know each other on a personal level."

An expert in international relations — particularly Soviet studies — Horn experienced what he taught.

He lived in Indonesia for a year working on his dissertation in 1967, and in Malaysia for a year in 1983 on the Fulbright scholarship. He traveled to the Soviet Union in 1979 for an International Political Science Assn. conference. A world map on his living room wall has clusters of pins denoting places he has visited.

He was no accidental tourist.

"We never put much money into our house," Judy said. "We used [the money] to travel."

He might not have put all that much into his house, but he put everything into his home.

"I don't know anyone who is a more model father," said Kit Machado, fellow CSUN professor and friend of 20 years. "He is devoted to his kids and it shows."

When his children played soccer, Horn rose at 5:30 a.m. every Saturday to set up goal posts at Winnetka Park with Sidwell, a league commissioner in the American Youth Soccer Organization. Horn was a deputy commissioner. In 1987 Horn formed the Valley United Wings club team.

Amy Hunter, a freshman on the UC Santa Barbara team, played for Horn on the Wings for three seasons.

"When I came to the team from a rival Simi Valley club, here I was, this new girl who knew maybe one person," Hunter said. "He went out of his way to make me feel comfortable and safe. He'd work with you individually and if you had a bad practice or got annoyed at another coach, he'd call you at home and say, 'Are you OK?' He was like a father to all of us. Whenever he was around, it seemed like everything would be all right."

Hunter lives in the UCSB dorms with Horn's daughter, Laura. Three other friends and former Horn players — Heather Gorman, Kris Bassler, who also plays for the Gauchos, and Kim Costantino — attend UCSB.

The archetypal coaching father, Horn coached his three children on youth soccer teams since the oldest, Jeff, 23, was 6. Chris, 21, and Laura, 19, each started playing soccer when they turned 5 and Bob coached them in AYSO leagues at Winnetka Park.

He also coached his sons in Little League baseball, but Judy said: "Girls' soccer was his main love."

Jeff and Chris both played soccer for Chatsworth High. But as Laura neared high-school age, the lack of a girls' soccer program hit home.

Horn went into action.

"He and others were active in getting L.A. Unified [School District] to approve a girls' soccer program," Judy said. "It was hard to believe there was no program. They had all sorts of excuses — no field space, no referees, no coaches. But whenever Bob could, he would talk to the Chatsworth principal. [Five] years ago, they finally approved it."

It was not a one-man effort, but Horn was a prime mover.

"I feel he was responsible for getting City soccer to happen," Sidwell said. "He wrote letters to the principal, made phone calls downtown, did a lot of work. I think [City girls' soccer] still would have taken place [without Horn], but it would have been two or three years later."

Horn took over the Chatsworth program in its second season, 1989-90, Laura's first year. He asked Sidwell to assist him and Steve Berk, the Chatsworth faculty coach of record.

The Chancellors won the City title that year. And the next.

Hirsch, the teaching assistant, often would drive the ailing Horn from CSUN to soccer practice.

"He put just as much into soccer as he did into his work," Hirsch said.

In Horn's second season, his symptoms became more pronounced. He began to fall while standing on the sidelines and soon was forced to ride around in a motorized three-wheel cart he could operate with his hands. He lashed a Mikhail Gorbachev doll to the front of the vehicle and called it "The Gorbymobile."

"That was fun," Horn said.

"What? Mowing down people?" said Judy, laughing.

Horn used a bullhorn to amplify his failing voice, but his condition deteriorated rapidly.

"By the time the championship game came around [in January, 1991], he didn't want anyone to see him," Sidwell said. "He was looking pretty bad. He was down on the sidelines at Birmingham High, but he had his wheelchair facing away from the stands."

He also had used his motorized wheelchair in the classroom. For a year, his CSUN students had picked him up at home and taken him to school so he could lecture, and many of them gathered in the hospital when Horn was in the intensive care unit for a month in February, 1991. The model United Nations continued.

Finally, unable to breathe or swallow, he opted to go on the ventilator at the end of February, 1991.

"He had been a participant all his life," Judy said. "Now he went to being an observer, watching his kids graduate from school and play sports, that sort of thing."

"The respirator isn't great, but it beats the alternative," Horn said.

The squat, blue metal box sits behind him on an end table. Horn sits in a nearby easy chair, looking every inch the professor, wearing a comfortable gray sweater, a shirt with a collar and a bemused, inquisitive gaze. A long plastic tube is affixed to his throat, methodically filling his lungs with air, breathing for him with the consistency of a metronome.

A gastrotomy tube — the gtube for short — is connected to Horn's stomach, feeding him a nutrient formula and medicine, and he requires round-the-clock care. A voracious reader, he finishes a book every two days with the aid of an electronic page turner he controls with a headband that senses his eyebrow movement. A small soccer ball sticker adorns the headband.

Judy said he loves to go to bookstores and attend church every other week, though he cannot venture out of the house often.

Horn is kept up to date on the Chancellors' progress this season by Sidwell. They are favored to win their fifth consecutive title, and Horn recently gave Sidwell a message for the playoffs.

"'Don't mess up and lose our first City championship,'" Sidwell said.

Chances are, they won't.

The Chancellors' closest match this season was a 4-0 victory over playoff-bound Granada Hills, and in seven matches, Chatsworth has outscored opponents, 54-3. The toughest match of the season? A 1-1 tie against the alumni in December. Horn wanted to attend but couldn't because of cold weather.

There are plenty of things he no longer can do.

"But, compared to what I can't do, I can do things that are important like love, feel, think, communicate, read and write," he said.

There is one other thing Horn *can* do. When someone incorrectly guesses a letter or word he is trying to say, his left eyebrow moves slightly downward and his lips, surrounded by a bushy salt-and-pepper beard and mustache, curve upward. His brown eyes sparkle.

Bob Horn smiles when he says no, as if forgiving the world for not being able to keep up with him.

Los Angeles Times
November 21, 1993

HE CHOOSES TO 'FIGHT THE UNBEATABLE FOE'

by Scott Harris

Bob Horn is a retired political science professor and he still has that professorial look. His hair is short and turning white, his beard more salt than pepper. His eyes are brown and compelling. A smile often curls the lips.

The amusement is reassuring, for though his features may be pleasant, looking at Bob Horn takes some getting used to. The disease known as ALS (amyotrophic lateral sclerosis) has robbed him of all but the slightest of physical movements — an arch of the eyebrows, the direction of his gaze, a tiny lift in his legs. He is unable to speak, eat or breathe without assistance.

A tube the diameter of a garden hose extends from his windpipe to a ventilator, which sits on an end table beside his easy chair in the living room of the Horns' Winnetka home. "The vent" inhales and exhales with a steady rhythm.

Bob Horn talks with his eyebrows; any movement means "yes." Bob and his wife, Judy, converse in a code, using the alphabet laid out on a grid.

"One, two, three, four..." Judy says. Bob raises his eyebrow; the letter is on the fourth row. "P,Q,R S,T" Judy says. Bob signals but Judy isn't sure. "Is it a T?"

Indeed it is. Judy guesses at the word. "The?"
Bob says yes.

***

Sometimes he talks with his feet. The disease may have deformed them, but because he still has some movement in his legs, he is able to nudge a special "mouse" rigged to his personal computer. The software enables him to scan the alphabet. Not unlike Judy, it offers "word prediction."

Bob Horn thus tapped out a letter to me last month. He was responding to a column about a woman's decision to end her terminally ill brother's life with a lethal dose of morphine.

"I am a supporter of legalizing euthanasia," he wrote. "In recent months, I have read and seen numerous reports about people with ALS who have ended their lives or sought to...I have become increasingly interested in the issue of doctor-assisted suicide. (In fact, I was offered that option by a physician at an earlier stage of my disease.)"

He proceeded to describe how, after 2 years on a ventilator, he finds life to be very much worth living. He enclosed some articles he had written for the newsletter of his church, Northridge United Methodist.

He tells of how he was moved by a TV news report on doctor-assisted suicide in Canada. Three people with ALS were considering the option — and all could still eat and talk. None was on a ventilator.

"I certainly don't mean to be judgmental," Bob wrote. "...I am not saying that I am in any way `better' or more courageous because I chose to go on living in spite of the disease."

He pointed out that the symptoms of ALS vary dramatically among patients. "For instance, one of the women in the report has a lot of pain, while I never have." And he well remembers the early stages of the disease: "As I have told Judy, for me `getting this way was worse than being this way.' You start dropping things, falling, having trouble swallowing, and losing your voice. This deterioration is, as you can imagine, quite depressing.

"Finally, the decision of whether to go on life support is an intensely personal one, I think. I made the right decision for me, but that doesn't mean it's for everyone.

"All that said, I would still like to talk to those people in the report. What would I say? Simply that `there is life on a ventilator'...I am an admirer of Don Quixote; I can identify with his willingness, as sung in `Man of La Mancha,' to `fight the unbeatable foe.' So be it."

Bob Horn loves to read and write and considers himself fortunate that he can still do both. He wears an athletic sweatband for reading. Inside it is a sensor that, when triggered by his eyebrows, activates a page-turning apparatus. On this day the subject was Shakespeare. Often he reads journals concerning the former Soviet Union — his specialty as a professor at Cal State Northridge.

If Bob Horn taps out G-O on his Macintosh, word prediction offers him the choice of "Gorbachev."

There are so many times, I told him, that I struggle for the right word.

"Any writer," he said with his eyebrows, "would love word prediction."

Then he grinned.

***

The impression that Bob Horn gives is that he wants his life to go on simply because he has done such a good job of living it. His home reflects the love of his wife and three children, now grown. His memories are rich with world travel and the simpler joy of coaching youth soccer.

He wrote his church columns several weeks ago, but there is a Thanksgiving quality about them. He expounded on the value of humor. He spoke of the importance of friends and family.

He knows that his slow way of talking, letter by letter, can have a certain dramatic effect.

"I think the real story," he said with Judy's help, "is about Judy."

Los Angeles Times
December 7, 1993

WITH LETTERS LIKE THESE, WHO NEEDS DRUGS?

by Scott Harris

...there is just one other letter I'd like to share.

This one concerns an article that appeared the weekend before Thanksgiving about Bob Horn, a former Cal State Northridge political science professor who has been left almost completely paralyzed and on life-support by amyotrophic lateral sclerosis (ALS).

Horn, using a special computer, had written in to explain that, while he believes that euthanasia should be legalized, he still finds life worth living. His body may have failed him, but his mind, heart and sense of humor are very much alive.

I interviewed him with the help of his wife, Judy. Bob doesn't speak; he moves his eyebrows, spelling out sentences in code.

Many people say Horn, who specialized in Soviet affairs, is an inspiration. He inspired this from Mark Romano of Glendale, a former student.

What your article didn't mention is how many of his former students are regular visitors at the Horns' even now. Bob and Judy are just that kind of people.

A note on the side: shortly after the attempted coup that nearly toppled Gorbachev, a group of friends were discussing Yeltsin's inevitable rise...The consensus was that it was a good thing that Yeltsin had preserved the nascent democracy. Horn's response has been borne out by events three years down the road, articulated with that "dramatic effect" of which you spoke: "W-h-a-t m-a-k-e-s y-o-u t-h-i-n-k t-h-a-t Y-e-l-t-s-i-n i-s a d-e-m-o-c-r-a-t?

He has a great mind and a great heart to match his great character and will.
For me, this is much better than drugs.

Los Angeles Times
December 31, 1993

HORN CAN'T SPEAK, BUT COACH'S MESSAGE IS LOUD AND CLEAR

by Kennedy Cosgrove
Special to *The Times*

Editor's Note

Times staff writers have provided a personal reflection on the 1993 area sports scene, chronicling the events and people that most affected them and offering an inside look at how reporters do their jobs. Today is the first of three days of those remembrances.

Nearly a year ago, I wrote a story about a soccer coach. His name is Bob Horn and he suffers from amyotrophic lateral sclerosis — commonly known as Lou Gehrig's Disease. In January, I learned about Horn, the former Chatsworth High girls' soccer coach who helped found the City Section girls' program in 1988. He had been an excellent coach, a renowned expert in Russian studies, a popular political science professor at Cal State Northridge for 22 years and a devoted husband and father of three.

Bob Horn, everyone told me, was the type of man who sucked the marrow out of life, not by yelling and screaming, but by caring. He was the type of man who invited his students to come to his house for barbecues. He was the type of man who rolled out of bed at 5:30 a.m. on Saturdays to set up soccer goal posts for his kids. He was the type of man who phoned his players at home if they had had a bad day at practice, just to say, "Are you OK?"

"He was like a father to all of us," said a former player. "Whenever he was around, it seemed like everything was all right."

When I first met Bob, the man who had traveled all over the world — teaching learning and exploring — he was physically unable to move any part of his body except his eyebrows, and, very slightly, his right leg. He communicated in painstaking fashion, one letter at a time, by raising his eyebrow as his wife, Judy, called out the desired letter.

I sat in their Northridge home while Bob (with Judy's help) told me about his choice — not an easy decision — to go on a respirator in February of 1991, rather than die. As happens with every ALS sufferer, the nerve cells that control muscular movement deteriorate. The ability to talk, move, eat and finally, breathe, are lost.

Some ALS sufferers choose to die rather than go on the ventilator. Bob's respirator sat next to his bed and rhythmically pumped air in and out of his lungs through a tube attached to his trachea.

I asked him about the ventilator.

"It isn't great, but it beats the alternative."

I asked him about all the things he could no longer do.

"Compared to what I can't do, I *can* do things that are important, like love, feel, think, communicate, read and write."

I asked him to tell me how he coped with the prison his body had become, asked him to put his mortality in full public view, to assess the value of his life.

And he did, with lively, humorous brown eyes and jokes he told letter by letter. He trusted me to tell his story, and I did, knowing it was worth the telling. I called the Horns the morning the story was published.

"It made his day, his month, his year," Judy said. She told me that friends from across the country had called, elated with the article.

Journalists generally are not in the helping business. Their job is to observe, interpret, report, not to make things better.

"I can't tell you how many positive and enthusiastic comments I received about your article," he said after I walked into the Horns' house two weeks ago. I hadn't seen Bob and Judy in 10 months. He had a new, improved computer that he was able to operate with his leg. His foot clicked the mouse, and he could use a special word processor program to write, which he did for his church newsletter. He could even print his documents.

"Good to see you, Kennedy!" he printed out.

He looked smaller, his body slightly more atrophied but his eyes were still warm and he could still smile.

I learned that Judy carried an added burden because their insurance no longer provided for the 16 hours of home nursing care per day, and she had to help pick up the slack.

"Judy wears her various hats as preschool director (her full-time job), nurse, bookkeeper, mother and wife, with grace, patience and understanding," Bob said.

She said it, of course, translating for her husband. Then she smiled at him. "Thank you."

But he also told her, "Show Kennedy the pictures."

Judy led me to his room, where the three photographs that accompanied my story were framed. She then pointed to a copy of the story I wrote hanging on his wall.

Before I left, I asked if the holidays were a time of poignant reflection for him.

"They are in a way more difficult because I am reminded of what I can't do," he said. "And at the same time more special because I am reminded of what's really important."

I nodded, and I picked up the piece of computer paper he had printed. "Good to see you, Kennedy!" it said.

I took it home and hung it on my wall, one writer's tribute to another.

Los Angeles Times
February 1, 1994

ORDEAL PUT THE PEDAL TO FAMILY'S METTLE

by Scott Harris

"This time," Judy Horn said, "our dogs alerted us."

Holly, usually a picture of calm, grew nervous. After the 3.8 aftershock hit early Saturday morning, the black Lab forced her way into Judy's room. Soon Judy was up feeding biscuits to Holly, Rex and the chronically skittish Butch.

Then Judy decided to check on her ailing husband. She was at Bob's side when the 5.0 aftershock hit at 3:20 AM, centered just a few miles north of their Winnetka home.

With one hand, Judy held on to Bob. With the other, she held on to his mechanical lung.

***

It's been two weeks and a day since the 6.6 haymaker sent us reeling. True, we don't know when the aftershocks will end. But as I took my own secret shortcut to work Monday, it was good to see that some of the fallen block walls were being rebuilt. Slowly, life seems to be returning to normal.

This also seems true for the Horn family — and normal for them is extraordinary.

Readers may recall Bob and Judy Horn. Bob is a former Cal Sate Northridge political science professor who five years ago was stricken with amyotrophic lateral sclerosis (ALS). Now virtually paralyzed by the disease, Horn survives with the aid of a ventilator — a battery-powered box that feeds air to his windpipe through a plastic tube. Prof. Horn still displays a sharp mind and an active wit with the help of a specially rigged computer or the coded movement of his eyebrows.

If the Jan. 17 quake was frightening for you, imagine what it was like for the immobile Bob Horn, whose mechanical lung was pitched to the floor and damaged. Imagine what it was like for Judy as she heard the ventilator alarm, signaling that Bob wasn't getting any air.

"I don't think I had time to go into the apprehension and fear," Judy says, "Because I had so much to do."

Judy and Bob, fortunately, weren't alone. Their 22-year-old son, Chris, was at home, as was a nursing attendant. So was Judy's 77-year-old mother, Marion, who'd shuffled in from the cold of Buffalo, N.Y., for a visit, only to come down with the flu.

The others made it through the quake without harm. They focused their attention on Bob.

First they disconnected Bob's broken "vent" and hooked up a device known as an "ambu bag" — a manually operated device that pumps air into his lungs.

This wasn't the only concern. Earlier that week, Bob had developed a bronchial infection that required the suctioning of fluids from his throat. With the power knocked out by the earthquake, they resorted to a portable, battery-powered suction device that provided only minimal help.

Bob's breathing became so difficult that Judy hooked up the device to an oxygen tank. For close to an hour, Chris used the "ambu bag" to keep his father alive. Judy dug through the books and memorabilia that had fallen in the den to retrieve Bob's wheelchair, with the portable ventilator attached.

Chris tried to explain his father's ordeal.

"He's helpless all the time," Chris said. "And when you run into something like an earthquake, when people who are not sick are helpless, it magnifies his helpless feeling.

"I was scared. My mom was scared. But that has to be shoved aside to make sure he gets through it...It was amazing what my mom was able to do."

Friends pitched in as well. A neighbor shut off the gas line. Mario Hernandez, a nursing assistant who has been with the Horns for three years, left his own damaged apartment in Reseda to check on the Horns. Chris' friend Ben Turner also showed up. Together, Chris and Ben were able to lift Bob into his wheelchair and place him in the van for a trip to the hospital, Humana West Hills.

Judy Horn has nothing but praise for how the hospital's doctors, nurses and attendants reacted to the crisis.

With Bob in the hospital, the Horns turned to chores at home. Broken pipes had flooded part of the house. A block wall was down in the back yard. Like so many people in the Valley, they were living without power, gas and water service.

"We're really, really lucky," Chris said. "There are people a lot worse off than we are." Judy's mother, who had always said she hoped to experience an earthquake on a California visit, headed home with a heck of a story to tell.

Last Friday, 11 days after the 6.6 quake hit, Bob came home from the hospital — just in time for a big aftershock.

Judy says they've learned a few lessons. Now Bob's ventilator is strapped to the table by a bungee cord. And his portable ventilator is close at hand.

***

Judy Horn tends to focus on the silver linings. One of the nice things about the Northridge earthquake, she says, is that old friends from all over the world have checked in to see how they're doing.

Sometimes, these calls have a certain poignancy. The other day, the Horns received a call from one of Bob's old frat brothers. They'd been out of touch for such a long time that he wasn't aware of Bob's illness.

But this friend, and all the others, would be happy to know that Bob's wit survived the quake just fine.

Talking with eyebrows, Bob says there is only one reason he went to the hospital.

"I couldn't deal with the clean-up."

Los Angeles Times
November 24, 1994

BOB HORN SPEAKS VOLUMES, BUT QUIETLY

by Scott Harris

Got a letter from Bob Horn a few weeks ago. Not a long letter, but it was packed with news, opinions and inspiration.

Now, I appreciate all my correspondence, for even hate mail stokes the glow of moral superiority. But Bob Horn's letters are special, and not only because he tends to be flattering.

Bob let me know he was moved by a column about "the blind fellow" — AIDS patient Mario Ceremano. "I was intrigued by his feeling of isolation," Bob wrote. Quickly shifting topics, Bob, a retired Cal State Northridge political science professor, expounded on a piece concerning the financial woes of the CSUN athletic department. He had kind words for Athletic Director Bob Hiegert, then added: "By the way, I have long favored dumping football."

Finally, Bob commiserated with my close-but-no-cigar lamentations concerning the Nippon Ham Fighters, my fantasy baseball team. "I can sympathize...because my team, the Slugs, on a very different point scale, ended up third, one point out of second and two out of first."

Many of you, especially those who lack a proper appreciation for fantasy baseball, may wonder why anyone would find inspiration in these words. But, as always, you have to consider the source.

This being Thanksgiving week, it was high time to drop in on the Horns.

***

His younger brother, Tom, has flown in from Pittsburgh, PA. His sister, Ethel, came down from Juneau, Alaska. The matriarch, Dorothy, was in from

Grosse Pointe, Mich. Today, Bob Horn and his wife, Judy, will be hosting 17 family members and friends for turkey and fixings.

I dropped by their Winnetka home on Tuesday. We sat in the living room, with Bob, as usual, leaning back in his easy chair, tethered by a plastic tube to his ventilator. The mechanical lung sat on an end table, inhaling and exhaling with a rhythmic wheeze.

Bob, virtually paralyzed, has been "on the vent" for four years. A fast-moving form of amyotrophic lateral sclerosis (ALS), also known as Lou Gehrig's disease, put him in a wheelchair and weakened him to the point that he was quickly losing the ability to talk, swallow or even breathe. His choice was death or life on the vent.

Bob Horn introduced himself to me last year by, as he would put it, "kicking out" a letter in response to a column concerning assisted suicide. Bob still has slight movement in his feet, and can write by operating a specially rigged computer mouse.

That led to a column about Bob's views on assisted suicide. He thinks it should be legalized, though it's not for him. A few months later, I checked in on the Horns again — and learned how the family survived the Northridge earthquake. Judy and their son, Chris, manually operated an "ambu bag" to keep Bob breathing, but a bronchial infection landed him in the hospital.

Bob was looking good Tuesday, better that I expected. An acquaintance had told me that Bob had lost much of the movement in his eyebrows. This was troubling, because aside from his computer, Bob "talks" with his eyebrows. The Horns rely on a code that employs the alphabet in a grid pattern. "One, two, three," Judy will say, and Bob will signal the row. Then Judy recites the letters, waiting for another signal. Fortunately, Judy usually needs just a few letters to guess at the word.

His eyebrows aren't as agile, but agile enough. His brown eyes are still attentive, darting from person to person. Often, a smile curls his lips. He silently shares in the laughter.

Judy, with Bob's prompting, filled in some of the highlights of the year. His old basketball buddy, elementary school teacher Martin Turley, visited often and got Bob out of the house more. They rode Metrolink and Metro Rail and stopped by the renovated Central Library. Bob, a Soviet scholar, wondered whether the library had a copy of his 1982 book, *Soviet-Indian Relations*. It did.

As a Father's Day gift, the Horns' three grown children — Jeff, Chris and Laura — took their dad to a Dodger game. It was a glorious day. The Dodgers won and Mike Piazza hit a home run.

Bob grinned and spelled out the significance. Piazza, it seems, doesn't just play for the Dodgers. He also plays for the Slugs.

***

"I'm a teacher," said the button on Bob Horn's sweater. He's now busy writing his second book, describing his ordeal with ALS. It takes him six hours "at best" to write a single-spaced page. The first 40 pages look promising.

Bob is a religious man, and I was curious about his opinion concerning efforts to allow prayer in public schools. He was precise in phrasing his answer. To him, "a moment of silence" — but not prayer — would be appropriate in the schools.

Only later did the irony strike me. This man has been silent for years.

But then I realized this wasn't true. Bob Horn isn't silent at all.

Los Angeles Times
January 15, 1995

Scott Harris Column

...Today being Reader Mail Day, there are just a couple of special letters from the files I'd like to share.

The first concerns Bob Horn, the former Cal State Northridge political science professor who is stricken with amyotrophic lateral sclerosis and now lives a productive, inspiring life attached to an artificial lung. Horn and his family have been the subject of a few columns, the most recent running on Thanksgiving Day.

Cheri Rae McKinney of Santa Barbara writes:

A few years back I was a "returned" student — a full-time political science major at the age of 32. Dr. Horn was the one professor who made all the difference to me...It was my good luck to be in Dr. Horn's class.

It only took a few weeks for me to realize I belonged in political science; I switched majors and never regretted my decision for a moment. I took Dr. Horn's Soviet Foreign Policy classes, and he talked me into taking his Model United Nations course. ...It was a wonderful class; at the end of the semester our entire class pitched in and purchased a beautiful new bicycle for Dr. Horn. (He had been riding a rusty wreck before that.)...

My heart aches to know about the deterioration of this vital man's physical condition, and I'm not at all surprised to know how active his mind remains...He is a teacher. A Great One!

Miracles, Signs and Significant Deeds
Joshua 10:12-14 & I Cor. 12:27-31
By Dr. David Richardson
Northridge United Methodist Church, Sept. 26, 1993

It was Jan. 10, 1945. General MacArthur and the American attack force lay off Luzon, ready for the retaking of the Philippine Islands from the Japanese. It was calm sea with less surf than anyone could remember. A typhoon had darted away at the last moment. American war correspondents humorously wondered if MacArthur could walk on water. To Filipinos this was no laughing matter. They believe to this day that the respite from the storm for the success of the mission was a miracle. MacArthur was the last man to disillusion them. As William Manchester comments, "He knew the power of myth in the minds of the islands' people. If they thought him capable of miracles, their conviction added a powerful weapon to his arsenal, one which his showmanship would polish."

What is a miracle? Is it showmanship? Is it a kind of grandiosity or megalomania? Rev. Asahel Munger, an early Methodist preacher in the frontier mission in the Willamette Valley, Oregon, was determined to work a miracle for the edification of the Indians. Acting on this passion he nailed his hand to a fireplace mantel. So impaled, he roasted to death on the mission hearth.

What is a miracle? Some T.V. evangelists use the motto, "Expect a miracle." That's what Rev. Munger did. He expected a miracle. Even Adolf Hitler expected miracles. Holed up in his bunker in mid April 1945, just weeks before the fall of Berlin, he received word from Goebbels about the death of Franklin D. Roosevelt. "My Fuehrer, this is the 'miracle of the House of Brandenburg' we have been waiting for, an uncanny historical parallel. This is the turning point predicted in your horoscope."

Miracles for some are the last hope against reality. Of course this leads to great cynicism. Mark Twain concluded that the only difference between a fact and a miracle is that fact requires proof and miracle relies on any kind of evidence. Hence, even at the end of the twentieth century we have reports of miracles such as a "holy tortilla" with the scorched image resembling the face of Christ, healings every week before our own eyes on television, and miracles of every description. I invite you to the metaphysical section of a bookstore for the details.

The question is, are these the miracles spoken of in our Bible? Is a miracle the cessation of the natural order, or the natural laws? Is a miracle the extraordinary? There was some great wisdom in the film, *O God,* when George Burns, as God, said, "Miracles are too flashy....The idea that anything connected with me has to be a miracle. It makes the distance between me and the rest of you that much greater."

I wonder if it is not true that the popular notion of miracle does distance us from God? Biblically speaking, the miracle is rather ambiguous. The Greek word for miracle, *thauma,* does not appear once in our Bible, nor does the Latin Vulgate use the term *miraculum* in the New Testament. The English word, "miracle," enters our text as a rendering of Hebrew or Greek words for such things as "wonder," "sign," "mighty works," "portents," and "significant deeds." The KJV uses the word "miracle" 37 times, the ASV uses it 8 times, and RSV 13 times. Goodspeed's translation, in keeping with the Vulgate, does not use the word at all. Roman Catholic theologian, Hans Kung, suggests it is better today for the most part to avoid the ambiguous word "miracle" all together.

The modern view of miracle as an interruption of natural law is not at all in keeping with the Biblical perspective. The writers of the Bible had no concept of natural law. Theirs was a prescientific world with no resemblance to ours. Hence when Joshua spoke to the Lord the sun and the moon stood still. This was no fact to be put to the proof as Mark Twain understood it. It stands as its own evidence, the report of the book of Joshua. One need not deliberate on the impossibility of the suspension of the whole universe, what it would mean to gravitation, or to the tides of the heat and cooling of the atmosphere, to understand the significance of the Amorites by Joshua. The sun stayed up long enough to accomplish this, just as the typhoon did not interrupt MacArthur's plans in the Philippines. A mighty act! Something to be grateful for.

St. Augustine tried to argue against interpreting miracles as being contrary to nature. The suspension of God's laws of nature is a contradiction in terms. Nature is nothing but God's will. We may catalogue the working of God, recognize the consistency and call this the laws of nature, but everything in nature is of God. Of course this perspective of Augustine has not always been followed. Even St. Thomas Aquinas viewed miracles as an interruption of nature.

The Apostle Paul downplays miracles as extraordinary. "God has appointed in the church first apostles, second prophets, third teachers, then workers of miracles, then healers, helpers, administrators, speakers in various kinds of tongues." It's fitting on this day Sunday School recognition that Sunday School teachers are more important in the scheme of things than miracle workers. But interestingly after he catalogues all these gifts of the spirit, he says I will show you something even more significant. Then he embarks on that greatest of all chapters in his work, the 13th chapter of I Corinthians, the love chapter. If I have all these gifts, even faith to move mountains, I am nothing without love. Nothing is greater than love, not even the miracle.

You see miracle must be put in its proper perspective. It is a sign, a significant deed but it is well within the scheme of things. In the Bible it is not something that distances us from God, but something that draws us closer to God.

It is non-Biblical works that cater more to the extraordinary as examples of miracle. Those of you reading Justo Gonzalez' book *The Story of Christianity* will read about the noncanonical works describing Jesus' life. As a child he breaks water jars of his playmates and throws them into a well. When they break into tears for fear of parental punishment, Jesus orders the water to return the jars unbroken. Jesus plays in tree tops like other children but he doesn't have to climb up, he simply orders the tree to bend down and he sits on it while it returns to its height.

While there are elements of such things in the Bible, the Bible does not fancifully view miracles. Yes the happenings may seem strange to our modern scientifically informed world view, but the Bible was not written with science in mind. It should not compete with science. Christians should not be trying to replace science in our schools with the Bible's world view. What the Bible is showing is signs from God, significant deeds. It gives us a way of looking at things that affirms God's presence in all that is, God's presence in all that happens. There is no distinction between nature and non-nature. God is not relegated to the unknown, the mysterious, the unnatural. All great things, significant deeds are of God. They are miracles.

Hence Russell Ogg who suddenly lost most of his vision due to diabetic retinopathy was able to rebound from the depression this caused him after catching sight of a hummingbird in the periphery of what vision he had. He went on to become one of the foremost photographers of these dramatic colorful birds. His biographer said, "Who can explain how miracles happen? Who can explain birth and rebirth or an awakening of spirit and mind? Who knows why or how a new self is born in a man because he suddenly saw a hummingbird?"

Miracle! Can you see the nature of miracle? As presented in our Bible it is something that brings us closer to God rather than something that distances us from God. Miracle is a sign, a significant work. It is not outside nature or contrary to nature, for nature is God's will. Above all it is love. The signs, portents, and mighty deeds point to God's power. We can rely on that. Above all we can rely on God's love.

What is a miracle? Perhaps this personal note from Bob Horn will help us all understand this question. I received the following three articles while I was working on the sermon. They summarized it better than I could ever do.

Personal 1

By Bob Horn

The other night I saw a report on CNN's "Headline News" that left me disturbed and thinking. It was about the controversy surrounding the issue of doctor-assisted suicide in Canada. Now that is a complex, disturbing, and thought-provoking issue in its own right. What personalized it for me, though, was that the three people the report profiled who all wanted to end their lives were all suffering from the same disease as I am, ALS. Moreover, its impact was intensified by the condition of the patients. With varying difficulty, all could eat and talk and none was on a ventilator.

I certainly don't mean to be judgemental, especially not after Maria's July 25 sermon. I am not saying that I am any "better" or more courageous because I chose to go on living in spite of the disease. This is the case for at least three reasons in addition to the ones Maria discussed. First, the symptoms of ALS vary dramatically from patient to patient. One person's experience with the disease is no guide to someone else's. For instance, one of the women in the report has a lot of pain while I never have. Second, I greatly sympathize with those people who are in the earlier stages of the disease for, as I have told Judy, for me "getting this way was worse than being this way." You start dropping things, falling, having trouble swallowing, and losing your voice. This deterioration is, as you can imagine, quite depressing. Finally, the decision of whether or not to go on life support is an intensely personal one, I think. I made the right decision for me but that doesn't mean it's for everyone.

All that said, I would still like to talk to those people in the report. What would I say? Simply that "there is life on a ventilator." Is that kind of life any good? That depends on what you compare it to. Compared to being "normal" the list of frustrations and "wants" is endless. Compared to being dead it's great! I suppose the bottom line is what you do after going on the vent. I am fortunate in that I love to read and to write and those I can still do.

One other thing about choosing to go on the ventilator: Where there is life, there is always hope. In the meantime, I am an admirer of Don Quixote; I can identify with his willingness, as sung in "Man of La Mancha," to "fight the unbeatable foe." So be it.

Personal 2: Coping

By Bob Horn

Some people, including Judy, have asked me how I cope. (I should ask the same question of her.) I hope part of the answer was made clear in my "Personal" article: I simply enjoy life in all its richness, diversity and complexity. Specifically, I have some personal thoughts which may or may not be relevant to anyone else.

Why me? At first, I agonized over that question. It isn't very productive, however, and it consumes a lot of emotional energy. Moreover, I eventually discovered what seems to me to be the logical answer to the question: Why not?

Fair? Of course it isn't fair. But then neither are some of the things that have happened to other members of this congregation or drive-by shootings of young children or Bosnia or Somalia. The list goes on.

Robbed, gyped, short-changed? You bet! After all, I was only 45 when I was diagnosed with ALS. Lots of living left to do. Lots of plans. On the other side of the coin, did I really have any room to complain? I had a wonderful wife, three terrific children, a career (college teaching) I had found both challenging and enormously rewarding, plus I had traveled widely and coached youth soccer for countless years. All things I loved. No regrets. And yet, I suppose it's human nature always to want more. I know I do. Result: Still an unresolved issue.

What is to be done? (Title borrowed from Lenin.) Fortunately, it's only my body that has turned to mush. I still have an active, if usually mundane and sometimes downright banal, mind. The following have been keys to my continued positive outlook:

1. Reading. I am enjoying the opportunity to do "recreational" reading there was never time for when I was teaching. I read almost as much and almost as widely as Dave! Everything from Russian history to world and Asian politics and novels of all kinds.

2. Keeping up with my professional fields of specialization. I still get several journals, both in hard copy and via computer.

3) Writing. I did a lot of writing when I was teaching — a book, monographs, articles and reviews — which I greatly enjoyed. Now, thanks to Dave and Maria (and all of you), I have been able to continue writing.
4) Humor.

To be continued. . . .

Personal 3: Clanging Cymbals? Not!

By Bob Horn

This is the final part of the "Personal" trilogy. It continues the discussion begun last time. The title refers, as you will see, to number six below.

4. Humor. For example, I have a calendar with lyrics from country-western songs; most are corny and some really tickle my funny bone. One that I have saved and taped on my wall puts my situation into perspective for me: "I can't decide whether to kill myself or go bowling."

5. Adaptive technology. Some of you have seen my electronic page turner which I operate with my eyebrows via a sensor in my headband. It has been indispensable. Recently, I also obtained a new computer with fantastic new programs; I am now able to do all the word processing functions I used to. And with my foot! It's actually fun!

6. Family and friends. I have saved the most crucial factor in my ability to cope for last. I simply don't think it would be possible without your love and support. My immediate family has, of course, been extraordinary in their patience, understanding, and encouragement. It has not been easy for them. Our extended family, the closest of whom live in Denver, has been supportive in a myriad ways; for example, my brother, a psychiatrist living in Pittsburgh, has become quite adept at finding professional meetings on the West Coast and then adding on a few days here.

For friends, let me use the example of the people of this church. Your love and support has been extended to Judy and me in literally countless ways. There has been practical help such as a roof, driving (and fixing) the van, food, financial support and keeping the books, legal advice, and more. Just as important has been the moral support, including always uplifting visits from Dave and Maria, prayers, cards, notes, letters, words of encouragement, our outstanding worship services and our wonderful music especially harps, bells and our marvelous choir. (Speaking of the choir and its soloists, I was overwhelmed by both the dedication and the beauty of the Mozart piece a few Sundays back.)

As Paul wrote to the church in Corinth, "If I speak in the tongues of men and of angels, but have not love, I am a noisy gong or a clanging cymbal." Well, no gongs or cymbals here! You are the instruments and reflection of God's love and I am continuously uplifted by you. You demonstrate that, as Paul further wrote, "Love bears all things, believes all things, hopes all things, endures all things."

Thank you.

October 1995

Dear Friends,

Back in July, the Worship Committee of our church, Northridge Methodist, asked Judy and me if we would be willing to do the sermon for our annual Laity Sunday in October. Perhaps incautiously, we said yes.

Since my public speaking skills are nonexistent — if my would-be book gets published, wouldn't I be great on the talk show circuit?! — we decided that it would make more sense for Judy to deliver it and me to write it rather than vice versa. In fact, Judy delivered it twice, at both services that Sunday.

The enclosed result, "Hurdles and Hurdlers," is our heartfelt thanks to each of you. You truly have been hurdlers. Thank you.

With love and appreciation,

Bob and Judy

HURDLES AND HURDLERS

Judy and Bob Horn
Northridge United Methodist Church
Laity Sunday
October 15, 1995

These are Bob's words:

They call him "Mr. Cub." He was on the National League all-star team nine times and was twice voted the league's Most Valuable Player. He was also the first African American on the Chicago Cubs. He is Ernie Banks and he is a member of the Baseball Hall of Fame.

Ernie had outstanding skills and it was a pleasure to watch him play. In retrospect, however, what impresses me even more than his ability is his attitude. He had an unparalleled enthusiasm and love for the game. One afternoon at Wrigley Field, he said, "It's a beautiful day for baseball. Let's play two." Think of it. An unscheduled doubleheader!

I think "playing two" is a perfect analogy for my situation. I am playing the second game of an unscheduled doubleheader. I almost died in early 1991. That's when I made one of the best decisions of my life: I chose to be hooked to a ventilator. I couldn't speak or move but, thanks to a machine and some tubes, I could breathe and eat! As I told Pastor Dave at the time, I felt re-born. Despite my limitations, it was good to be alive. It still is. I am enjoying playing my second game.

There are several factors that explain my ability to cope with Lou Gehrig's disease, to play two as Ernie Banks said. Far and away the most important is YOU — Judy's and my church family, our friends from soccer, the university, and other walks of life, and our families. My story, which is also Judy's story, is just as much about you as it is about us. In fact, without you, there wouldn't be a story. We have seen God working through you. We have experienced literally countless expressions of God's love from you. In the words of a beautiful song from the wonderful musical, Les Miserables, "To love another person is to see the face of God." In you, we have seen the face of God, felt His presence and been touched by His love. You have sustained us.

What is particularly amazing about you people who have been so supportive is that whenever I reached a turning point in the progression of the disease, a new obstacle, someone would suddenly appear with a solution. Every time I was confronted by a new hurdle, one of you became a hurdler. God does indeed work in mysterious ways sometimes. The more I think about it, though, the more the ways don't seem so mysterious because they have been so consistent. Shortly after a problem would pop up, a person or a group of them with an answer would, too.

There have been many hurdles along the way and, fortunately for Judy and me, just as many hurdlers. We would be here the entire day if I recounted them all. Let me give you just a few examples.

My physical deterioration was extremely difficult for me because of the new limitations it imposed almost weekly. When I could no longer ride my bike nor drive a car, students of mine volunteered their assistance to get me to and from the university. When hauling me in and out of a normal car became too awkward and I was pretty much confined to a wheelchair, friends offered to have their van converted to make it accessible for my use. It brought me here this morning. When I began to lose my energy and stamina, colleagues at the university were able to find ways to lighten my teaching load. When I had trouble writing, a friend volunteered to be my right hand. And, as my voice weakened, she came up with the alphabet chart that I still use for communicating. Her help has become increasingly valuable over the years and I recently bestowed upon her a huge new title. She is now my Administrative Assistant and Literary Advisor. Impressive, isn't it? Incidentally, I also have a Director of Player Personnel for my fantasy baseball team — which finished in first place this year. As you can tell, I am big on titles, probably because I am not big on salaries.

Two prominent examples of the right people appearing unexpectedly on my horizon at the right time were my "computer gurus," Jan and Diane. They were exceptional. As the ALS progressed and left me too weak to raise my hands to the keyboard, along came Jan. I hate to think of how many hours he must have put in on my behalf designing, from scratch, a program that would enable me to type with my eyebrows. He was never satisfied and was constantly working to improve his original creation. Every time he came up with a new version, he would spend a whole evening with me in my study having me test it and make suggestions. Then he would go home and work on it some more. We finally settled on version six or seven! Jan's dedication, especially for someone who was volunteering his time, was just remarkable. His invention worked beautifully for three years until my weakening eyebrows made it too difficult for me to use. To say that I was discouraged would be a vast understatement. And then, voila, along came Diane, a specialist in adaptive computer equipment. She was the one who noticed my slight leg movement and then designed and installed a terrific system which utilizes that tiny movement. As a result, for the last two years I have been typing with my foot which, as a friend pointed out to me, is quite appropriate for a retired soccer coach.

When I felt I needed some sort of creative outlet, a means of communicating what I had been reading and what was in my head about the collapse of the Soviet Union and the end of the Cold War, you allowed me to start writing regular articles for the church newsletter. Three and a half years and more than 50 articles later, I can't begin to tell you how big a favor you did for me. As long as you don't rebel, I would like to continue.

A final example. One of the major burdens the family of an ALS victim faces is financial. Sooner rather than later, most patients are going to require some level of nursing care. How much depends on the amount of responsibility the spouse, if there is one, is willing and able to assume. How skilled depends on the stage of the disease. Before I went on the ventilator, I needed only part-time, relatively unskilled help; once hooked to the vent, however, I required around-the-clock skilled care. This is extraordinarily expensive even if insurance picks up part of the tab. Seeing this financial nightmare looming imminently, a group of our friends decided to do something about it. Without our involvement, they established a fund which still exists to this day. It has been of enormous assistance in defraying the high cost of my care. Since we lost our nursing coverage two years ago, it has been absolutely critical.

There have been studies which show that social support, as opposed to social isolation, positively correlates to longevity in terminally ill patients. This doesn't surprise me at all. From my own experience, I can testify that social support like Judy and I have received also positively correlates to QUALITY of life. That is even less surprising.

You cannot imagine what your love and support have meant to us. In words and deeds, you have enriched our lives under these difficult conditions. Through you, we have been blessed by God's love.

Let me close by suggesting that each of us, when confronted by any kind of adversity, has a basic choice. We can either cope or mope. This choice was put perfectly by Calvin and Hobbes in an August strip. Calvin is bemoaning the fact that summer is almost over. "Soon school will start," he complains. "No more freedom, no more long days outside, no more fun." Hobbes replies, "Well, let's go make the most of the time we have left." "Nah," says Calvin, "I've reserved the rest of the month for moping."

Coping with ALS, while not my idea of fun, is obviously doable but I would dread having to face it alone. In fact, without your love and support, I would dread even moping.

Thank you.

Amen.

Selected, Annotated Bibliography

Listed and annotated below are the "Top 20" books that have, in a variety of ways, contributed to my thinking about living with disability and terminal illness. Actually, there are only 19 listed because one book, about a person's struggle with ALS, proved to be unfindable in the post-earthquake Los Angeles library system. Not listed are the almost countless relevant articles from newsletters, newspapers, magazines, and journals.

Anderson, Terry. *Den of Lions. Memoirs of Seven Years.* New York: Crown Publishers, Inc., 1993.

This account by the former hostage of his captivity in Lebanon is an incredible story of courage and faith in enduring almost seven years (2,454 days to be exact) of inhumane and degrading treatment. Some of the most moving parts of the book are Terry's poems and the sections written by Madeleine, then his fiancee and now his wife.

Ashe, Arthur, and Arnold Rampersad. *Days of Grace. A Memoir.* New York: Alfred A. Knopf, Inc., 1993.

This is the late tennis great's very moving autobiography. It deals with everything from his tennis career to his struggle against racism to his involvement in various political and social issues. However, Arthur's major focus is on his battle with AIDS. Although the disease eventually claimed his life, he definitely was a winner.

Beisser, Arnold R. *Flying Without Wings. Personal Reflections on Being Disabled.* New York: Doubleday, 1989.

As a young man of 25, Beisser was struck down with polio. The book is about how he managed his life after that — dealing with his disability, becoming a psychiatrist, getting married and maintaining an active practice in psychiatry. Its main thrust is an excellent discussion of coming to terms psychologically with disability.

Browning, Norma Lee, and Russell Ogg. *He Saw a Hummingbird.* Midland, MI: Northwood Institute Press, 1978.

Russell was a photographer until the progressive disease of diabetic retinopathy eventually left him blind. He was in despair until, with the tiny bit of sight that remained, he observed equally tiny hummingbirds next to the patio of their home. What followed is a remarkable story of not only how he became a renowned photographer of hummingbirds but also how he regained purpose and meaning in his life.

Chenevert, Basil J. *Taking Hopelessness Out of Helplessness.* Detroit: J.R. Printing, 1989.

This booklet is full of practical suggestions to help paralyzed ALS victims on ventilators achieve a measure of independence and control in their lives. It is written by an engineer who was himself stricken with ALS.

Cousins, Norman. *Anatomy of an Illness as Perceived by the Patient. Reflections on Healing and Regeneration.* New York: W. W. Norton, Inc., 1979.

This is a fascinating story of Cousins' successful battle with a disease of the connective tissue thought to be nearly incurable. It is about the link between the mind and body in fighting illness, particularly the value of laughter. He makes a strong argument for the significance of this link.

Cousins. *Head First. The Biology of Hope.* New York: Penguin Books, 1989.

If negative emotions have a deleterious impact on health and well-being, isn't it rational to think that positive emotions have opposite physiological effects? This book amasses a great deal of evidence in support of that proposition. It is based on the 10 years Cousins spent as a member of a task force researching this question at the UCLA School of Medicine.

Hanlan, Archie J. *Autobiography of Dying.* Garden City, NY: Doubleday & Company, Inc., 1979.

Hanlan kept a tape-recorded diary from the beginning of his struggle with ALS. Most of the book is comprised of this diary, an insightful and often poignant progression of his thoughts about death and dying. Another valuable part of the book is the postscript written by Mary Hanlan, his wife. Entitled "Living with a Dying Husband," it powerfully portrays the toll a disease like ALS takes on a spouse.

Hine, Robert V. *Second Sight.* Berkeley: University of California Press, 1993.

A professor of history at the University of California, Riverside, Hine dealt with diminishing eyesight from an early age until he was almost 50 when he went completely blind. An operation restored his sight 15 years later. In the last chapter he compares the worlds of the sightless and sighted and discusses some aspects of disability in general in a thought-provoking way.

Jackson, Edgar N. *Understanding Grief. Its Roots, Dynamics, and Treatment.* New York: Abingdon Press, 1957.

Written especially for pastors counseling the bereaved, Jackson's book contains many insights for the rest of us. It is based on numerous case histories.

Kaye, Dennis. *Laugh, I Thought I'd Die. My Life With ALS.* Toronto: Viking, 1993.

This is a superb book. It is realistic yet inspirational. Kaye was stricken with ALS at the relatively young age of 29 and his story is one of courage, loaded with humor and keen insights. It is also, in part, an eloquent appeal for increased public awareness, and hence greater funding for research, of ALS. The middle section of the book is a practical guide for victims of the disease.

Kubler-Ross, Elisabeth, M.D. *On Death and Dying.* New York: Macmillan Publishing Co., 1969.

This seminal work examines attitudes toward death and dying focusing particularly on the stages the terminally ill work through. It also explains what the dying can teach others, including doctors and nurses, clergy, and even their families. It is based on interviews with more than 200 patients.

Lindbergh, Anne Morrow. *Gift From The Sea.* New York: Vintage Books, 1955, 1975.

This book is old, short, written particularly for women and says not a word about disability or terminal illness. Yet, I found much in her insights and wisdom that is relevant to my life and situation.

Malcolm, Andrew H. *This Far and No More. A True Story.* New York: Times Books, 1987.

At age 40, "Emily Bauer" was stricken with ALS. This is the story of how this physically active woman, a psychologist and mother of two very young children, and her husband dealt with her disease and its rapid progression. She ultimately decided that she couldn't live such a severely limited life. Much of the book focuses on her struggle to be taken off the ventilator and allowed to die. She eventually succeeded.

Rabin, Roni. *Six Parts Love. One Family's Battle with Lou Gehrig's Disease.* New York: Charles Scribner's Sons, 1985.

The subtitle tells all. Written by a daughter about her afflicted father, it is a story of love, support and courage in the face of a disease that severely tests entire families at a time. This family coped admirably. I found this book much more positive and uplifting than Malcolm's, which I thought was depressing.

Siegel, Bernie S., M.D. *Love, Medicine & Miracles. Lessons Learned About Self-Healing from a Surgeon's Experience with Exceptional Patients.* New York: Harper & Row, 1988.

I found both of these books by Siegel fascinating and very helpful in the early stages of my disease. With a progressive disease like ALS, however, Siegel's approach is ultimately unsatisfactory. Although he denies it, there is a strong implication that you are responsible for your illness and that if you can't heal, it's your fault. (See Spiegel.)

Siegel, Bernie S., M.D. *Peace, Love & Healing. Bodymind Communication and the Path to Self-Healing: An Exploration.* New York: Harper & Row, 1989.

This book, too, draws its examples mainly from Siegel's cancer patients. One aspect of the books that I still like is their focus, as with Cousins and Spiegel, on the interaction between the mind and body in dealing with serious illness. To me, the point of that interaction is coping, not necessarily physical healing.

Spiegel, David, M.D. *Living Beyond Limits. New Hope and Help for Facing Life-Threatening Illness.* New York: Times Books, 1993.

This uplifting book focuses on the interaction of the mind and body in coping with serious illness. Disease can't be wished away but one's mental outlook can substantially affect the quality of life and maybe even its longevity. His empirical evidence is based mainly on his experience with cancer patients but is equally applicable to other diseases.

White, Michael, and John Gribbin. *Stephen Hawking. A Life in Science.* New York: Penguin Books, 1992.

This is a very readable biography of the renowned British scientist who has had to cope with ALS for all of his adult life. Since he is less than a year older than I am, that means for over 30 years! What he has accomplished in spite of the disease is awesome and truly inspiring.